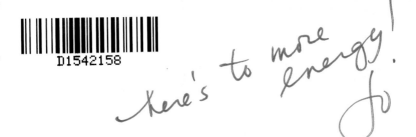

here's to more energy!

Jo

Praise for Dr. Jo's®

REBOOT

"*Jumpstarting a new you can be a tough task, but Dr. Jo® shows you how... with her characteristic humor and practicality.*"
Brian Wansink PhD, Author of *Slim by Design* and *Mindless Eating*

"*Want more energy? Dr. Jo delivers with sound science, can-do spirit, and hundreds of sensational tips for the way you think, move, sleep, and eat. I love it!*
Marlene Koch, RDN, New York Times bestselling author of *Eat What you Love Everyday: 200 All-New Recipes Low in Sugar, Fat, and Calories*

"*This terrific book is packed with little life-changers: simple ideas that make a huge difference. Three weeks after incorporating just a few of the basic strategies, my weight is down, my energy is up, and I'm ready to take it to the next level. Thank you, Dr. Jo!*"
New York Times bestselling author Joni Rodgers

"*Personal, positive, powerful! Dr. Jo® gets it --with real science, practical solutions and wit. Her energetic and candid approach can REBOOT your mindset, food choices, and lifestyle for a healthier and more productive you!*"
Roberta L. Duyff, MS, RDN, Author of the best-selling *Complete Food and Nutrition Guide* from the Academy of Nutrition and Dietetics

"Dr. Jo's REB*OOT is a tour de force! Dr. Jo once again weaves important health and wellness information into an easy-to-read clever handbook. In Reboot, Dr. Jo shows us exactly how what we eat can result in our dwindling energy and productivity. Highly recommended.*"
Dr. Janet Brill, nutritionist and author of *Blood Pressure DOWN* (Three Rivers Press, 2013)

(more on the next page...)

Other Books by Dr. Jo

Dr. Jo's No Big Deal Diet
How to Stay Healthy & Fit on the Road
Eat Out Healthy

Dr. Jo's®

REBOOT

how to power up your energy,
focus, and productivity

Dr. Jo Lichten, PhD, RDN

Nutrifit Publishing

Published in Orlando, USA
DrJo.com

Library of Congress Control Number: 2014920120

Publisher's Cataloging-in-Publication
(Provided by Quality Books, Inc.)
        Lichten, Joanne V.
            Reboot : how to power up your energy, focus, and
        productivity / Dr. Jo Lichten, PhD, RDN.
            pages cm
            Includes bibliographical references.
            ISBN 9781880347997
            ISBN 9781880347980

            1. Health.   I. Title.

        RA776.L53 2014   613
                                QBI14-600184

ISBN 978-1-880347-99-7

Acknowledgments

I'd like to acknowledge the many talented women who helped me get this book to press. I couldn't have written this book without PJ Dempsey, my content editor. She took my initial 500 page research-heavy manuscript (can you say, "Oy vey?") and helped me organize it and then chisel it down to a fun, but still educational reading book. Then, Joni Rodgers, my creative editor and consultant, made sure Dr. Jo's voice was still there after all the editing. She's also the one that, throughout the multiple cover revisions, finally said, "Why don't we put Dr. Jo on the cover?" Check out this wise and wonderful woman (and award winning author) at www.jonirodgers.com. Thanks also to Elizabeth Piarote who designed my cover, (Meg Salvia (copy editor), Charla McKinsey (photographer), and Stephanie Prosonic (typesetting).

Second, thanks to my sweeties! My husband, John, and daughters, Ali and Melissa, were always there to support me with kind words of support, input, and patience. For more than two years of intense research and writing they would ask, "What are you going to do today?" and I would respond, "I'm gonna finish my book today." Except for one day, this did not happen...but they still never doubted me or this project. These three very special people energize my life!

Table of Contents

ALT
Discover an Alternate Food Pattern 53

1

The REBOOT Solution

I knew I was awake. I just couldn't wake up.

C'mon, my brain begged my body. *Listen. Take notes. You're missing it.*

I focused on my foot, one toe at a time, thinking if I could just wiggle that foot, I would be able to shake off the scary weight of this…whatever this is. I was more than simply tired; I felt like I was almost in a trance.

Thirty years later, as a Ph.D. nutritionist and registered dietitian who has dedicated thousands of research hours to the science behind human energy, I know that it was a full-blown case of fatigue involving weakness, lack of energy, and exhaustion. It settled over me like a cement blanket when I was in college, and it had the power to immobilize me at times. I'd be sitting in class, eyes wide open, straining to pay attention, and gradually realize that I was paralyzed, the way we are when we're wrenched from a deep sleep.

Fatigue has many causes – it's different for each of us. For me, it started when an eating disorder turned my life inside out. I dropped 40 pounds just before I went off to college, where I promptly gained it back and stacked on another 25. (They had an "all you can eat" cafeteria plan, and I followed instructions. That's the kind of girl I am.) Over the next few years, my weight fluctuated wildly in that 65-pound range as I zealously embraced one fad diet after another, and my energy level continued to plummet. Mind you, this was all while earning my bachelor's degree in nutrition, which only goes to prove that knowledge is *not* power. Intellectually, I understood the nature of the beast, but that lingering fatigue kept me helpless to make the necessary changes.

All that changed after graduation when I worked on a research study that examined the possibility that regulating blood glucose levels would help people suffering from Meniere's disease (a chronic condition of dizziness and ringing in the ears). My job was to instruct people to eat in a way that regulates glucose (the fuel our brain runs on), adjust the calories to make sure they didn't lose weight (so weight wasn't a conflicting factor), and collect data regarding incidence and severity of the Meniere's episodes. But most of the time, these people just wanted to talk about was how much energy they had.

"My husband can't believe it's me!"

"I used to fall asleep at my desk at about 2:00 in the afternoon, but now..."

"After all these years, I finally have the energy to do things like..."

Hiking. Playing with the kids or grandkids. Reading without falling asleep.

My ears perked up. I couldn't even imagine what it would feel like to bound out of bed in the morning and take on the day with such joy and animation. My head started spinning with questions: What creates human energy? Why do some people have it and others don't? How could these participants have more energy even if they didn't even lose weight? Could *when* you ate food really impact energy? I immediately stopped dieting and began thinking of food as fuel for my body and my brain. Within a week I felt better; within a month I was feeling great! And the excess weight started coming off without hunger (and has stayed off for 30+ years). Finally, with my new, energized body, I had the patience, focus, and mental energy to dedicate my career to understanding the other parts of the puzzle regarding human energy so I could help others.

Another light bulb flashed during a master's degree course on neurophysiology at Virginia Tech, part of which focused on the dynamics of sleep – another major piece of the energy puzzle. What most people don't appreciate is the fact that the secret to a refreshing night's sleep is quality, not quantity. And, yet, how many of us share the bed with a pet or a snoring partner? Every nighttime interruption, whether you fully awaken or not, can impact your energy the next day – even if you were in bed for a full eight hours.

Realizing that stress, emotions, and old habits can get in the way of good intentions, my doctoral dissertation from Texas A&M University focused on the difficult process of how we make health changes. After years of university teaching, I spent much of the 1990's developing and presenting full-day seminars. As a trainer for one of the world's largest business training companies, I taught stress management to business executives. In addition, I developed continuing education courses for health professionals on diet, movement, sleep, and stress management. During this time I researched how we might better identify and work with our individual circadian rhythms to manage a nightshift schedule, jet lag, seasonal affective disorder – as well as a work schedule that requires us to drive to work in the dark and return home without ever seeing the sun. I learned how even something as simple as our thoughts and worries can exhaust us. Stress itself isn't the culprit (heck, some stress is actually healthy), but the way in which we respond to it can impact our energy levels, and our response is something we have the ability to change.

After decades of this diverse experience, I currently spend my time helping people manage their personal energy – keynoting at conferences, writing books and articles, and coaching C-suite business executives at the Human Performance Institute in Orlando, FL. Now I'd like to help you have more energy than you've ever imagined.

MEASURING THE COSTS OF FATIGUE

"I'm so tired," a client tells me.

"How tired?" I ask, because that could mean tired like *stayed up too late with a good book* tired or *partied like it's 1999* tired. Or it could be true fatigue.

Like pain, fatigue is difficult to measure objectively, but researchers are trying to figure it out. For now, we can gauge fatigue only through questionnaires and checklists. One thing we know for sure is that fatigue doesn't feel good, and its ramifications have far-reaching effects. Fatigue negatively impacts health, safety, work performance, family life, social relationships, and life satisfaction. It's also very costly to the corporate bottom line:

● **Fatigue interferes with daily activities:** Fatigue decreases reaction time and influences accuracy in making decisions. Fatigued people tend to have reduced attention spans and impaired memory; they may also be impulsive and prone to misunderstandings.

- **Fatigue increases accidents and errors:** Fatigue increases accident risk through slowed reaction time and reduced attention and processing speeds. A 2012 report by the World Health Organization identified fatigue as one of the causes of medical error and injury in healthcare.

- **Fatigue increases absenteeism and missed work:** In the large, three-year Maastricht Cohort study, fatigue was related to both short-term and long-term absence from work.

- **Fatigue is costly to business:** When people go to work but aren't feeling well ("presenteeism," as opposed to "absenteeism"), it hurts work performance. And, it turns out that the price of this loss of productivity is even more expensive, maybe as much as four times more, as the outright medical costs. That means that fatigue may be more costly to businesses than sleeping problems, high cholesterol, hypertension, obesity, and other chronic pain.

MY GOAL IN THIS BOOK

I want to help you get out of bed in the morning without dragging, take on your day's most tedious tasks without nodding off, and get home at the end of the day with enough residual energy to enjoy the people and things you love. First, we'll take a brief look at the physiology of fatigue, then we'll break out some simple ideas you can put into immediate action.

As we REBOOT, you'll learn:

- Where "energy" comes from and why some of us have it, and others don't

- How thoughts and worries work to exhaust you – and how to stop them

- Why some meals energize you while others drag you down

- Why it's okay (necessary, in fact) to give yourself a break, how often to take breaks, and which types of breaks work best

- How movement impacts energy (plus more than 100 fun ways to get moving)

- How and what to eat and drink before, during, and after working out to recharge your body and maximize that sweat equity

- How you can experience better quality sleep without spending more time in bed

- How often (and how much) to eat for energy, without packing on the pounds

- How to work with your circadian rhythm to manage shift work and jet lag

- Why even slight dehydration can depress your energy, mood, and attention and even bring on headaches

- The pros and cons of caffeine, energy drinks, vitamins, and supplements

- Best meal and snack options at home, in restaurants, and on the road

- Simple damage-control strategies to initiate when you're crashing

My bleary-eyed younger self would never have imagined that friends and colleagues would approach me almost every day with the same question: "Dr. Jo, where do you get your amazing energy?" With all the demands and opportunities of life in a super-charged world, it's the hottest topic in my field of expertise: What is this precious natural resource we call *energy*, and how can we get more of it? For a few lucky people (I'm not one of them), it comes naturally.

For the rest of us, there's REBOOT.

WHY REBOOT?

We all wish we had more hours in the day, and I don't have a magic wand to make that happen. I actually have something better: the real science and practical action items that will enable you to generate more energy to get more accomplished in a day. Once you REBOOT your energy, you'll feel as if more hours were magically added to your day. In addition, you'll reap the many benefits of increased energy, including:

- Wake up feeling refreshed

- Remain alert (even during boring meetings or long drives)

- Stay motivated to work when you need to
- Have a positive attitude that shows in everything you do
- Feel energized after eating (without being goosed by the busy person's best frenemies: caffeine and sugar)
- Keep your weight within a normal range with little effort
- Enjoy your down time (without the need for drugs or alcohol)
- Delight in hobbies, friends, and other interests
- Keep debilitating stress at bay

There are medical conditions – some of them serious – that may cause fatigue. So check out some of the causes listed in Appendix A and consult your physician for a full evaluation. That said, here's a familiar refrain I hear all the time: "My doctor couldn't find anything wrong, but I still feel like I've been hit by a bus." This can be incredibly frustrating. The good news is that even if all known medical reasons are ruled out, there's still much you can do to REBOOT your lifestyle and say goodbye to feeling exhausted, unmotivated, and overwhelmed – just like you'd reboot a computer that's on the fritz.

PC users are familiar with the three-finger salute they give their computers, simultaneously holding the CTRL, ALT, and DEL keys to shut down programs, and then RESTART the system. In many regards the human body is no different; some of us need an occasional REBOOT to fine-tune our bodies, so we feel more focused, energized, and more productive. Using these same steps (CTRL, ALT, DEL, RESTART), here's how REBOOT works:

CTRL – CONTROL YOUR CIRCADIAN RHYTHM

Inadequate sleep impairs coordination, performance, and reaction time as much as being intoxicated. That's right: driving tired can be just as dangerous as driving under the influence (and negatively affects our work performance as well). Sleep is critical to maintain optimal energy, personal relationships, health, weight, and work productivity. You might be able to fool yourself momentarily with a temporary energy boost from caffeine or sugar, but (as the song says) you end up "writing checks your body can't cash." Medications might help you get to sleep at night, but there can be ill repercussions, and feeling rested it isn't just about how many hours you spend in bed.

In the CTRL section, you'll learn how the sleep cycle recharges both the body and brain and how you can maximize the effect simply by strategically setting your alarm in order to awake feeling energized. We all have a natural circadian rhythm, programmed within every cell in our body, which determines when we are the most productive and when we should take a break to recover energy. The good news is that it's possible to reset the body clock for managing jet lag, nightshift work, working late, or even the occasional *party like it's 1999* moment.

ALT – DISCOVER AN ALTERNATIVE FOOD PATTERN

A microwave oven needs electricity. Your car needs gas. And your body needs—c'mon, I know you know this one that's right! *Food.* Food creates the energy we need to perform work, including mental and physical activity as well as maintaining emotional stability. Calories are often considered "bad guys," but in fact, calories are simply a measurement of energy. Calories are required for life and critical for peak performance, and it's only when we eat too many, too few, or the wrong types of calories that we run into problems.

Think back to the last time you went too long without eating. Perhaps a meeting ran through your usual lunchtime or you had a close connection between flights. Going too long without food not only makes us hungry, but also tired, irritable, impatient, shaky, and unable to concentrate. On the other hand, a large meal with a lot of calories doesn't provide us with bounds of energy. *Au contraire*, it leaves us feeling sluggish and lethargic. Clearly, fueling for peak performance isn't simply about eating adequate food or enough calories; it's about eating the *right* food, at the *right* time, in the *right* quantity.

The ALT section explores an ALTERNATE food pattern that will help you get more energy from food while trimming excess body fat. We'll also discuss how much fluid we need to stay hydrated as well as longer-lasting energy-amping alternatives to the temporary boost we get from sugar and caffeine.

DEL – DELETE NEGATIVE STRESS

You're on your way home after a long day at the office, mental gears shifting between that last email you sent and what's for dinner, what the kids are up to in the back seat, and the lane change that will take you to your exit.

Suddenly, a horn blares from your blind spot. Brakes shriek behind you. Instantly, every fiber of your being – from eyebrows to sphincter – is in that driver's seat, behind that steering wheel, focused, responding. Wide awake.

In that split second, your body released the hormone adrenaline which promptly set off a chain reaction, increasing blood pressure and heart rate in order to get sufficient oxygenated blood to the muscles needing to respond quickly to this danger. The body also releases additional glucose into the bloodstream to provide the extra fuel that's also needed. Adrenaline is called the "fight-or-flight" hormone because it helps us fight or flee danger – real or perceived.

This reaction can be lifesaving, but experiencing it over and over again is actually life threatening – and exhausting. Yet, many of us put ourselves through this exhausting fight-or-flight reaction hundreds of times in a day in response to a wide range of situations, most of which are nowhere near as touch-and-go as a traffic incident.

The DEL section offers strategies on how to delete stressful thoughts and actions so we can save the fight-or-flight reaction for the true emergencies.

RESTART – USE MOVEMENT TO RESTART THE ENGINE

We all know why we *should* exercise, and we're all familiar with the most frequent excuses for not doing it, including lack of time, interest, or equipment. That's because most of us are stuck in the mindset that we need to go to the gym – but we don't! We tend to think about the chore of *exercise* instead of focusing on the joy of *movement*. What's cool about movement (aside from the fact that it just sounds like a lot more fun than exercise, don't you think?) is that while movement *expends* energy (since it burns calories), it can actually *expand* our personal energy by building muscle mass to bump up your metabolism and increase muscle strength and endurance. But we don't get stronger by simply moving more. It's a two-step process: first, exercise/movement breaks down the body; then we build it back stronger with the optimal refueling foods and drink to help you get the body you want.

In the RESTART section, you'll find doable solutions for movement that even the busiest of people can use, more than 100 fun ways to move that don't involve a gym, and guidelines for incorporating small chunks of movement throughout the day to generate physical, emotional, and mental energy while meeting official exercise recommendations.

So now you know what to expect. Ready to REBOOT?

CTRL

Control Your Circadian Rhythm

"I don't get it," Sondra tells me. "I was a vegetable the whole weekend, slept all afternoon Saturday, and didn't get up until noon on Sunday. By Monday afternoon, I was exhausted again. How am I supposed to get through the week if two days isn't enough to catch up on sleep?"

Catch up on sleep? She may as well try to lasso the moon while she's at it. That's not how sleep works. The key to feeling fully rested and healthy is to control your circadian rhythm both during the day and at night by: (1) paying attention to your sleep cycles, (2) resetting your body clock with healthy daytime and nighttime habits (so it's easier to fall asleep when you want to), and (3) using recovery breaks and powernaps to extend productivity.

Sondra doesn't need to be unconscious for twelve additional hours every weekend; she needs to spend her week consciously cultivating blissful, productive, energy-boosting Zzzzzs so she can get out and have fun on her days off.

2

All About Sleep

Michael is always the designated driver. He takes it seriously because his brother was killed by someone driving under the influence. Michael has drummed it into the heads of his teenage kids: *you don't drink and drive*. He's the friend who won't let friends drive drunk. But he's about to walk out the door and get behind the wheel after a long night spent tossing and turning. He knows he didn't get as much sleep as he needs to face a long day at the office. What he doesn't know is that inadequate sleep impairs coordination, performance, and reaction time just as much as a blood alcohol level in the intoxicated range.

Sadly, many people consider it normal to feel so sleepy by midafternoon that they're fighting to stay awake. Then there are those who think that sleep is overrated and proudly wear their exhaustion as a badge of honor. While caffeine and carbohydrates may offer a temporary reprieve for sleepiness, it's impossible to completely compensate for the loss of sleep, and sleep is absolutely critical for maintaining optimal energy, personal relationships, health, weight, and work productivity. Getting adequate rest is more than spending a set number of hours in bed. To REBOOT your energy, you'll need adequate amounts of the *right type* of sleep.

THE MANY BENEFITS OF ADEQUATE SLEEP

Chances are, you already know that getting seven to eight hours of sleep is recommended. But don't just take this statement at face value. Research by the National Sleep Foundation via annual polls found that people say they function best when they get about seven to seven and a half hours of sleep every day. Unfortunately, these same polls indicate most people are about thirty minutes short of that. And, I'm betting it's even worse than that because people tend to report bedtime as when they get *into* bed, not the time they actually *fall asleep*. It's no wonder that about one third of us say we unintentionally fell asleep at our desk, on the couch, or behind the wheel in the past thirty days.

Sleep plays an essential role in keeping us healthy and success-ful. Sleep is critical for clear thinking, quick reaction times, and efficient problem solving. It also helps the body fight disease and recover from injury. Mom was right when she simply told us to go to bed instead of immediately reaching for medicine or sending us to the doctor. While I'm not suggesting you stop going to the doctor, let's face it: most of the time all we can do is rest and let the illness run its course. Adequate sleep helps you recover faster. The latest research indicates that chronic sleep deprivation may also be a major contributor for the increase in conditions such as diabetes, high blood pressure, depression, and even weight gain.

THE CONNECTION BETWEEN SLEEP AND WEIGHT

It's hard to REBOOT your energy when you're carrying around extra pounds. Sleep deprivation can increase weight in several ways:

- The longer you're awake, the more opportunities you have to eat. Because sleep deprivation makes high-calorie foods more enticing, you'll probably reach for sweets and salty snacks. This craving is something that can actually be viewed using functional magnetic resonance imagery (fMRI), as high-calorie foods stimu-late the reward areas of the sleep-deprived brain.

- When you're tired, you're more likely to be sedentary and avoid physical activity.

- Sleep deprivation adversely affects the secretion of two hor-mones: it increases ghrelin, which stimulates hunger and reduces leptin, which makes us feel full.

Getting a good night's sleep is just as critical if you're working at losing body fat. In one fascinating study, dieters lost the same amount of weight whether they were provided adequate sleep or were sleep deprived. But during the sleep-deprivation period, they lost more lean muscle mass and less fat.

RATING YOUR SLEEP HABITS

Now it's easy to rationalize and blame fatigue on unproductive meetings, mundane tasks, or boring TV shows. But the research is clear: quickly falling asleep during the daytime hours is indicative of inadequate sleep at night. A boring meeting will always be boring, but it shouldn't lull you to sleep.

Sleep latency is the term scientists use to measure how long it takes to fall asleep while lying in a darkened room. What it comes down to is this:

- Taking more than ten minutes to fall asleep during the day generally indicates normal alertness.

- Taking less than eight minutes to fall asleep is considered abnormal and means you need more sleep.

- Falling asleep in under five minutes or experiencing microsleep episodes (where you suddenly fall asleep or nod off for even a moment) while involved in a task is considered severe pathological sleep deprivation.

Some people mistakenly interpret the fact that they can fall asleep quickly as a sign of being able to relax easily, even though this is a clear indicator of sleep deprivation. Laboratory studies of people who fell asleep quickly found that increasing the time slept at night consistently increased the time needed to fall asleep during the day. Up to a point, the more sleep you get at night, the more alert you are during the day. Studies prove that even when one night's sleep is reduced by only one and a half hours, there's a 32% reduction in daytime alertness.

The Epworth Sleepiness Scale

The Epworth Sleepiness Scale is a well-researched tool to help you determine if you're getting enough sleep. Simply rate your chances of dozing during each of the seven sedentary situations listed below using the following scale and add up your scores.

Chances of Dozing:
0 = Would never doze
1 = Slight chance of dozing
2 = Moderate chance of dozing
3 = High chance of dozing

Score Each of these Situations:
_____ Sitting and reading
_____ Watching TV
_____ Sitting inactive in a public place (e.g. a theater or a meeting)
_____ As a passenger in a car for an hour without a break
_____ Lying down to rest in the afternoon when circumstances
       permit
_____ Sitting and talking to someone
_____ Sitting quietly after a lunch without alcohol
_____ In a car, and while stopped for a few minutes in traffic
_____ **TOTAL SCORE**

A score of 10 or more is considered sleepy.

CIRCADIAN RHYTHM

Because we live on a planet that makes one complete rotation on its axis every twenty-four hours, it's easy to assume that we've conveniently adapted to this environment by sleeping at night and waking up in the morning. Yet humans left in a windowless environment without clocks and allowed to eat and sleep as desired naturally adapt to a *nearly* twenty-four-hour cycle of sleeping and waking, referred to as a circadian rhythm. Scientists have long known about the master internal clock in the brain that maintains this pattern, but recently they discovered that every cell in the body also maintains this same *nearly* twenty-four-hour cycle.

The circadian rhythm is evident in more than the cycle of sleeping and waking; it also affects blood pressure, body temperature, stress hormones, and other bodily functions that fluctuate in a predictable pattern throughout the day. One such pattern concerns the hormone melatonin. (It's not just a supplement; our bodies produce it naturally.) Melatonin production goes up at night to promote sleepiness and decreases as morning approaches to make you feel more alert. What's more, remember being told when you were a kid that sleep was important to both your growth and getting better when you were sick? Well, that's true because the growth hormone that enables the body to heal and grow is most active at night. Not everyone's master clock is set exactly the same. Some of us like to get up early in the morning, while others like to sleep in. Yet, even with these differences, we humans are daytime creatures who tend to get sleepy during the night. This is why workers on the night shift have a harder time staying alert during their shift and have more health and weight issues than day workers. Any time we try to force the body to adjust to an abnormal circadian rhythm, there are consequences. While it is possible to *adjust*, realize that humans don't ever *adapt* completely to a nocturnal schedule.

SLEEP CYCLES

Within a twenty-four-hour circadian rhythm, the body experiences about sixteen ninety-minute cycles of alertness, both sleeping and awake. Let's begin by discussing the cycles that occur during sleep and how not getting enough sleep or the right type of sleep can majorly affect energy.

Sleep works like a tune-up or a major "defrag" for the brain. If you don't get enough of the right type of sleep, you can be a basket case all day long. Waking up on the wrong side of the bed or spending the day not being able to think straight might mean that you actually woke up on the wrong stage of a sleep cycle.

We sleep in chunks of time called sleep cycles, each lasting about ninety minutes. During a good night's sleep, we experience a succession of about five of these ninety-minute sleep cycles, one right after the other. During each of these sleep cycles, we experience both REM and non-REM sleep.

REM Sleep is the dream stage characterized by rapid eye movements. While it's possible to dream in any stage, dreams appear to be more vivid during REM sleep. Even when we don't remember dreams, we all likely dream. We know this from research in sleep labs; when people are awakened during this stage, they clearly remember their dreams. Getting enough of REM sleep is important to maintaining emotional stability and mood regulation.

Non-REM Sleep (most sleep is non-REM) is comprised of three stages designated by the electrical activity of the brain:

- Stage 1 occurs when you feel drowsy and drift in and out of consciousness. You might think you're awake but then suddenly forget what you were thinking about. In meditation, it is referred to as alpha stage because the brain emits alpha waves.

- Stage 2 is a slightly deeper stage of sleep where you spend roughly half your sleep time. During this time, the heart rate and body temperature decrease to prepare for sleep; muscles experience alternating periods of muscle tone and relaxation.

- Stage 3 is a very deep stage of sleep noted by slow-wave or delta brain waves. This stage is pretty much a semicomatose state with very little body movement. If you are awoken in this stage, you will be confused and groggy.

While all three non-REM stages are critical to rebuilding the body, the deeper stages (stages 2 and 3) also contribute to intellectual ability and memory. It's no mystery why you get sick more often and make more mistakes when you don't get enough sleep.

Anatomy of a Full Night's Sleep

At 11:00 PM, you close the book you've been reading, turn off the lamp on your nightstand, snuggle into fresh linens, and close your eyes. Soon, your mind and body are relaxing into Stage 1 sleep, and for five or ten minutes, you drift in and out of consciousness.

By 11:20, you're drifting deeper, to Stage 2: a light sleep in which your pulse slows and your body cools. You drift deeper, to Stage 3: deep, restorative sleep, during which your muscles, bones, and immune system regenerate and repair. Then you return to Stage 2.

After midnight, close to 90 minutes into your sleep cycle, you're dreaming in a light REM sleep. Your subconscious mind is sorting images and processing the tidal wave of input presented to your eyes and ears every day.

By 12:30 or so, you've completed the first ninety-minute sleep cycle and begun the second cycle consisting of stage 2, 3, 2, and back to REM. This is repeated throughout the night. If you sleep for six hours, you'll experience four ninety-minute cycles. This increases to five cycles if you sleep seven and a half hours.

Each ninety-minute sleep cycle is slightly different. While just 10% of total sleep time is spent in stage 3, most of this is during the early parts of the night. Although 20–25% of total sleep time is in REM stage, the time spent there is briefest in the first few sleep cycles, with most REM sleep occurring during the latter hours of sleep.

REM sleep is a lighter sleep, so it makes sense that we feel more energized when waking at the *end* of any ninety-minute sleep cycle, rather than in the *middle* during deep sleep. If you have time for only six and a half hours of sleep, consider getting up after six hours because you'll feel better waking from the light stages of REM sleep than the deeper sleep you'll experience if you continue into the next sleep cycle. This is especially true when you're sleep deprived. While most deep sleep is experienced in the first few hours, sleep deprivation changes the game, resulting in deep sleep continuing into the early morning.

The same holds true when sleep is constantly interrupted. Each time something wakes you up, the body slips out of deep sleep and has to start the sleep cycle all over again. It's like that Monopoly game card that sends you back to GO without collecting $200. In other words, with disturbed sleep, you spend the same amount of time in bed but without all the benefits.

REBOOT TIPS TO GET THE MOST OUT OF A NIGHT'S SLEEP

Remember, it's not just about getting the right hours of sleep; it's about making sure you get the right type of sleep. So:

- **Limit interruptions:** Get pets off your bed, and possibly out of the bedroom. Even if you don't awaken fully with their movements, it's likely you'll be knocked out of a deep sleep, so your body has to start that cycle all over again. This disrupts the delicate sleep-cycle balance and impacts how you function the following day. Unfortunately, we don't have as much control over our partner or kids, but helping them to get a good night's sleep will help everyone function at their best.

- **Get to bed early:** The best way to feel energized, alert, and healthy is to go to bed early enough to wake up naturally when your body says it's had enough sleep.

- **Reconsider the tone of your alarm:** Don't shock your brain awake. Instead, go with the softest sound that will wake you or an alarm that starts softly and increases in volume if it's ignored. You can also choose an alarm that combines sound with gradually increasing light to wake you naturally.

- **Consider the sleep cycles:** Before setting the alarm, take into account the ninety-minute sleep cycles and plan accordingly. There are sleep apps (including The Sleep Cycle, Sleepbot, and Sleep As Android) that wake you during the lightest level of sleep. Set it for the time you must wake up, and the alarm will wake you during your lightest stage of sleep *prior* to that time.

- **Skip the snooze button:** Get up immediately and resist the temptation to hit the snooze button because it could knock you back into a deep stage of sleep, especially if you're sleep deprived.

Perhaps you're wondering how to set the alarm to get the required ninety-minute sleep cycles when you haven't the foggiest idea how long it takes you to fall asleep. If you're having a hard time getting to sleep, it could be that your body rhythms are not aligned with the sun. Don't laugh; there's truth to this statement. Read on.

3

Reset the Body Clock

Nurse Nan (as her colleagues affectionately call her) heads up the graveyard shift in a busy emergency room, a mentally and physically demanding job that requires her to be wide awake and ready for anything from eleven at night until seven in the morning. "Why is it so much harder in the winter?" Nan asks. "I get the same amount of sleep I do in the summer."

The answer to her question happens to be one of my favorite words: *zeitgebers*.

Earlier, I mentioned that the circadian rhythm is *nearly* twenty-four hours. While some of us have cycles a little shorter than that (more women than men), on average, we're about twelve minutes *over* the twenty-four hours. That doesn't sound like much until you realize the ramifications of adding twelve minutes a day over even as little as a week. This means that if you were in a darkened room without any time cues on the first night and you start feeling sleepy at 11 p.m., the second night it wouldn't be until 11:12 p.m. On the third night, this wouldn't occur until 11:24 p.m., and on the fourth night, it would be 11:36 p.m. This extra twelve minutes a day in the circadian rhythm causes problems of less sleep each night, assuming you have to be up at the same time every day.

Luckily, in the real world of light and dark, we naturally use external cues to reset our body clock to stay closer to a twenty-four-hour schedule. Scientists call these external cues *zeitgebers*, German for "time-giver" or "synchronizer."

LIGHT

The most powerful zeitgeber to reset the master clock is light. That's why Nan has a harder time in the winter. It's a good idea to get at least thirty minutes of daylight every day (with appropriate sunscreen of course) to REBOOT the body clock back to a more appropriate twenty-four-hour schedule. But Nan doesn't get up for work until well after sunset.

Time in the daylight helps shorten or lengthen the circadian rhythm more closely to a precise twenty-four-hour schedule. If you have a hard time getting up in the morning, yet find yourself wired late into the evening, get outdoors during the early daytime hours (7 a.m.–2 p.m.) to help your body *shorten* the circadian rhythm back to a twenty-four-hour day. On the other hand, if you tend to fall asleep early in the evening, get outdoors during early evening hours (5–9 p.m.) to *extend* your cycle. If it's not possible to get outside, consider getting a light-therapy device for daytime reading. By the way, getting your daylight through a car or office window won't work, and midday light (2–5 p.m.) doesn't seem to have much effect in adjusting our cycles, either

DARK

The second most powerful zeitgeber is nightfall. When the sky turns dark, the pineal gland in the brain starts producing the hormone melatonin, which makes us sleepy. Unfortunately, most of us live in a place where life doesn't stop or slow down when it gets dark. There's TV to watch, work to do, email to answer, and other things that really *must* get done before bedtime. The light from these devices actually prevents the brain from producing melatonin, making it harder to fall asleep. When light enters the eyes, the signal travels to the master clock in the brain and turns off the melatonin production in the pineal gland.

WHAT'S YOUR CHRONOTYPE: MORNING LARK OR NIGHT OWL?

While melatonin production occurs each evening, the onset can vary by as much as six hours. Those with an earlier onset are referred to as morning larks. These individuals go to bed early, get up early, and perform their best and are most productive in the morning. Night owls would rather go to bed late and sleep in. Not surprisingly, night owls do better work in the afternoon and night and tend to manage night-shift work better than morning larks.

These different chronotypes can also affect health and weight. Morning larks tend to have lower resting heart rates, half as much sleep apnea, and lower body weights than night owls who stay up later. Night owls tend to eat fewer meals, fewer fruits and vegetables, more fast food, and more full-calorie sodas, and consume most of their calories during the latter part of the day. They also tend to be heavier. In addition, night owls tend to get less sleep, perhaps due to jobs and other commitments that don't permit them to sleep in.

Of course, not every job or societal expectation accommodates an individual's preferred chronotype. If you want to postpone melatonin production to stay up a little longer, or not wake up so early, get into daylight in the late afternoon or early evening (5–9 p.m.). If you have a hard time getting to sleep, get more morning light (7 a.m.–2 p.m.) and reduce the amount of nighttime light (including what is emitted from the computer, tablet, TV, and cell phone).

REBOOT TIPS FOR FALLING ASLEEP EASILY

When you need to reset that clock and increase melatonin production to be able to fall asleep without a lot of tossing and turning, try these tips:

- **Pick a bedtime and stick to it:** Don't go to bed at 9 p.m. on work days and stay up until 3 a.m. on your days off because it will screw up your body clock.

- **Practice a nighttime ritual:** Take a lesson from your parenting; we know that a nighttime routine (snack, brush teeth, change into PJs, read a story, turn out the light) helps kids get ready for sleep, so do the same for yourself. Turn off the TV and computer, dim the lights, and read a book. You may also find quiet music or a warm bath helpful.

- **Dim the lights:** Indoor lighting (including light emitted from TVs, computers, cell phones, tablets, and the blue suffuse aircraft cabin lighting) can delay melatonin production, reduce how much is produced, and shorten its duration. If you tend to wake up too early in the morning even though you're tired, turn off the evening lights even earlier to boost melatonin production. In addition, turn off the hall light and draw the blinds (consider using blackout shades). When traveling, carry binder clips to securely close the blinds. Use a very dim night light in the bathroom, if you must. Also, make sure your clock isn't emitting too much light. If so, unplug it. When you need to sleep on the red-eye flight, or when you just can't get the bedroom completely dark, consider wearing an eye mask.

- **Sleep in a cool room:** Both extremely hot and cold bedrooms can disrupt sleep. A cool room is recommended for a better night's sleep because it mimics the natural drop in your body's internal temperature that occurs during sleep. Pile on the blankets and put on your bed-socks, though, if you're too cold.

- **Keep it quiet:** Noise makes it more difficult to fall asleep and reduces sleep quality. Even if you think you're capable of sleeping through noise, you're not. With increasing noise, especially intermittent noise, your body responds by falling out of that deep, restful sleep and into a lighter stage of sleep. So, turn off the phone and use earplugs or a sound-soother machine (yes, of course, there's an app for that!) to block distracting noises.

- **Exercise regularly:** A recent survey by the National Sleep Foundation found people who exercised as little as ten minutes a day were more likely to report that they got a good night's sleep. They tended to fall asleep easily and experience more deep sleep. The more exercise they got (and the more intense the exercise), the better they reported their sleep, even with the same amount of sleep. The only caveat for exercising late in the evening is that it prevents *some* people from winding down.

- **Skip the nightcap:** Alcohol may help you to relax and feel sleepy, but it prevents long-lasting rejuvenating deep sleep. Even as little as one quarter of an alcoholic beverage decreased duration of sleep.

- **Avoid large meals and beverages before bedtime:** A small evening snack is fine (unless you experience acid reflux), but don't eat large meals two to three hours before bedtime. Drinking too many fluids after dinner will keep you awake running to the bathroom.

- **Check the medicine cabinet:** Talk with your physician and pharmacist about your medications. Certain meds (like decongestants) can prevent you from getting a restful night's sleep.

- **Avoid caffeine and nicotine:** Both are stimulants and lead to reduced sleep. Later in this chapter, you'll see how even one morning cup of Joe can be the culprit for insomnia.

- **Practice strategic napping:** Limit daytime naps to thirty minutes or less and avoid naps after 3 p.m., unless you work nights (see Chapter 4).

- **Write down your worries:** When thoughts and concerns make it difficult to fall asleep, jot them down. Then, each time your mind wanders in that direction, remind yourself that you've written it down, so you won't forget about it, and there's nothing you can do about it until the morning.

- **Use the bedroom only for sleep and sex:** Avoid watching TV or doing work in bed because these actions set up an association that signals your brain that the bed is not for sleep. If you can't fall asleep, get out of bed, sit in a chair, and read a book under a dim light until you feel sleepy (not an e-reader or tablet because that light will decrease melatonin production).

LIGHT THERAPY SOLUTIONS

If your body clock is out of whack, and daylight isn't available due to work hours, you can REBOOT your system with light therapy. Light therapy has been shown to be effective in relieving symptoms related to seasonal affective disorder (SAD), shift work disorder, and jet lag. Here's how it works:

Light is measured in lux. Living-room lighting has 50–200 lux, typical indoor office lighting has 300–500 lux, and daylight on a clear day measures about 50,000 lux. Light therapy involves shining bright artificial light (2500–10,000 lux) indirectly on the face (not directly on the eyes) for about thirty minutes to two hours (at the appropriate time) to improve sleep-wake quality and mood. Talk to your physician regarding recommendations of light devices that filter out harmful UV rays and have been tested to be effective.

Seasonal Affective Disorder

Seasonal affective disorder (SAD) is a real problem (it is more common in women) characterized by depressed mood, fatigue, longer sleeping patterns, weight gain, and carbohydrate craving during the winter. Incidence increases with increasing latitude; one study found that rates ranged from 1.4% in Florida to 9.7% in New Hampshire. Another study demonstrated that, in response to the approach of winter, melatonin secretion in people with SAD increased more than a half hour earlier at night, making them sleepy earlier in the evening.

If you're suffering from SAD and don't get much natural morning light, ask your doctor about using light therapy for one hour first thing in the morning. Because light has antidepressant properties, light therapy is often the treatment of choice for SAD. Light has a low risk of adverse effects. Many studies have shown it to be just as effective as antidepressants, and the response is often quick (half respond in as little as a week).

Shift Work Disorder

Humans are daytime creatures, yet 20% of the population works a shift other than a regular daytime shift. As many as one third of these night-shift workers experience a host of performance and health issues labeled as shift work disorder. These issues arise from staying awake all night, when the natural internal circadian rhythm wants the body to sleep, and attempting to sleep during the day during the circadian rhythm of alertness. Besides fatigue, symptoms include decreased attention to detail, slowed reaction time, attention lapses, reduced coordination, and compromised problem solving leading to increased injuries, errors, and accidents. Car accidents are more common on the drive home from a night shift, too.

Shift workers also have more health risks. They tend to be heavier than day workers. Not only do sleep-deprived individuals eat more, hormones including insulin, ghrelin, and leptin all have circadian rhythms that don't support eating at night. Gastrointestinal disease, such as peptic ulcers, GERD, and irritable bowel syndrome (IBS), are also more common in shift workers and are thought to be related to this disruption of the body clock. Night-shift workers have an increased risk for developing depression, heart disease, diabetes, and breast and colon cancer. In fact, the World Health Organization has stated that circadian disruption due to shift work is probably carcinogenic in humans.

Shift work tends to become more difficult as a person ages, and morning larks tend to have more problems adjusting. The impact of shift work on health increases with exposure, and it does not seem possible to improve one's ability to adjust over time, even with permanent night work.

REBOOT TIPS FOR MANAGING SHIFT WORK

The reality is that although it is not possible to ever fully adjust to shift work, there are some things that can be done to make this schedule more manageable.

- **Design an effective work schedule:** If you work eight-hour rotating shifts, it's best to rotate shifts in a clockwise direction. There's some controversy on how quickly the rotations should change. Because more consecutive days provide an opportunity to achieve synchronization, it's suggested that rapid rotation, such as working different shifts in the same week, should be avoided. Others argue that because the circadian rhythm can only be reset an hour or two per day, a rapidly rotating schedule is best because it minimizes time spent in a desynchronized state. If your workplace allows an option, find out which strategy works best for you.

- **Adhere to a strict sleep schedule:** Strict adherence to regular sleep and wake times, even on days off, can help you adjust to a consistent night shift. As much as possible, minimize noise and keep those sleeping hours sacred. Don't schedule appointments during designated sleep times.

- **Sleep in darkness:** Keep the bedroom very dark (again, blackout shades are helpful) because there's a strong association between a dark bedroom and length of sleep.

- **Consider when it's best to sleep:** Some shift workers prefer to sleep right *after* their shift, while others find more effective realignment when they sleep later in the afternoon, just *before* starting their night shift. If sleeping right *after* the shift, wear sunglasses that block out blue light on the drive home.

- **Use bright lighting during work shifts:** For a modest but significant circadian realignment, use bright lights at the appropriate time during the day and night. When sleeping right *after* the night shift, use bright-light exposure from 11 p.m.–3 a.m. and seek exposure to bright light after waking in the afternoon. When sleeping right *before* the night shift, it helps to use bright-light exposure between 3–7 a.m. and get some bright light upon returning home.

- **Practice strategic napping:** The longer you're awake, the sleepier you will be. Therefore, it helps to nap right *before* work to decrease the desire to sleep during the night. Brief naps (15–20 minutes), if permitted, *during* the shift can also improve reaction and cognitive function in the second half of the night shift.

Jet Lag

Jet lag is also a circadian-rhythm disorder. A Conde Nast survey found that 93% of respondents suffered from symptoms of jet lag, including fatigue, difficulty concentrating, muscle soreness during the day, and not being able to sleep fully at night after a long-haul flight. Because the gastrointestinal tract has a circadian rhythm, jet lag can cause stomach problems, constipation, and diarrhea. Jet-lag symptoms also tend to be worse and last longer the more time zones you cross, especially after travel in an easterly direction. It takes about a day to recover for each time zone crossed.

REBOOT TIPS FOR MANAGING JET LAG

The following tips may appear contradictory, but remember that every trip is different in terms of length and time traveled and time zones crossed. What works for one trip may not work for another.

- **Prepare in advance:** Go to bed earlier several days prior to an eastward trip, but go to bed later prior to a westward trip, to catch up to the time of the place to which you're traveling.

- **Keep to your hometown schedule:** Because it takes roughly one day to recover for each time zone crossed, try to approximate your hometown schedule, especially if the trip is brief.

- **Adopt the local schedule right away:** Though light and dark are the most effective zietgebers and the easiest way for you to slide into the new time zone, other cues such as meals and other activities specific to the time of the day help to reset the body, too.

- **Use sleep aids:** It's difficult to get to sleep when it's nighttime, and your body clock still thinks it's daytime. Pack and use earplugs, eye masks, and sound soothers to assist in getting to sleep.

- **Use light:** The sun or another source of bright light is effective in resetting the body clock. Bright lights in the early morning tend to shorten your day, so you'll feel sleepy earlier. Bright lights around dusk will lengthen your day, so you can feel more alert past your usual hometown hour.

- **Consider melatonin:** Melatonin is highly effective in preventing jet-lag symptoms. For best results, choose a lower dose with immediate release rather than slow release (see below for detailed dosage information).

- **Tips for traveling east:** When traveling on a night flight, use an eye mask to get as much sleep as possible on the flight. Then, on the next day, stay outdoors or in bright light in the afternoon or early evening (around your hometown bedtime) to help reset your body clock to a later time. When traveling on a day flight and desiring to adopt the local schedule, avoid sleeping on the flight. To get to sleep on the local time, avoid bright lights in the evening (even TVs and computers) and use an eye mask. Be sure to get some bright-light exposure first thing the next morning to effectively shorten your body clock.

- **Tips for traveling west:** When traveling west on a morning flight, take a nap. This will prevent you from falling asleep too early in the evening at your new location. Then, stay outdoors or in bright light in the evening (around the time of your usual hometown bedtime), but avoid it the next morning to lengthen your body clock.

Melatonin Supplements

The Natural Medicines Database rates melatonin supplements as "likely safe" and "possibly effective" for short-term use. Melatonin supplements do seem to help with jet lag. However, melatonin is a hormone, and it hasn't been studied on a long-term basis, so it shouldn't be taken on a regular basis. As with other sleep aids, rebound insomnia has occurred when some people stopped taking melatonin. What concerns me the most is that, as with every other supplement, the FDA offers no oversight regarding its safety or efficacy. Many supplements have been found either to not have the dosage specified on the label or to contain contaminants.

The typical dose for melatonin is 1–3 mg, but timing is more important than dose. If trying melatonin, consider that immediate-release melatonin is better for difficulty falling asleep, while sustained-release melatonin is better for difficulty staying asleep.

Melatonin supplements should be used along with light (at the right time) for synergistic effect. One study found that evening bright light cancelled out the effects of melatonin even when sub-jects used as much as 5 mg. Because the body produces melatonin naturally, when having trouble getting to sleep, follow the healthy nighttime habits mentioned earlier in this chapter.

CAFFEINE'S HALF-LIFE AND SLEEP

We all know that too much caffeine can make it difficult to fall asleep, but even one morning cup of coffee can have the same effect. While the alerting effects of our favorite caffeinated bever-age are felt fifteen to thirty minutes after we drink it, it takes about twenty-four hours or longer for the body to eliminate the caffeine in a single cup of coffee. Caffeine is a drug, so the body needs to eliminate it, and how fast or slow this happens is measured by its half-life. Half-life is the amount of time it takes for the body to eliminate *half* of what's in the bloodstream. For caffeine, this is about four hours, but it can vary from person to person. It tends to be shorter in smokers and as long as twenty-four hours in women who are pregnant or taking oral contraceptives.

While we often hear that a cup of coffee has 100 mg of caf-feine, that measure is for an 8-oz cup, and most of us drink from 12–16-oz mugs. Also, some coffee makers and specialty coffee shops extract more caffeine from the coffee beans, resulting in even higher caffeine content. The caffeine in black tea varies based on how long it's been brewed, but an average cup contains 50–100 mg. Green tea, generally, has half the caffeine of black tea, and a 12-oz can of caffeinated soda has 50–75 mg of caffeine. There's a full list of foods, beverages, and medications with their respective caffeine content at the end of this chapter.

Assuming the average half-life of four hours, let's calculate the length of time it takes for a cup of coffee to leave your body. If you drank a venti-sized cup of coffee (400 mg caffeine) from Starbucks at 6 a.m., 200 mg will still be circulating in the body four hours later at 10 a.m. At 2 p.m., another half of what remained gets eliminated, so there's still 100 mg in your bloodstream. At 6 p.m., another loss of half results in 50 mg, and at 10 p.m. there's still 25 mg of caffeine in your body. We all have different sensitivities to caffeine, but even as little as 25 mg of caffeine can affect sleep. Now imagine that in addition to your morning cup of coffee, you drank more servings of caffeinated beverages later in the day. What amount of caffeine would still be in your bloodstream at bedtime? If you're having trouble sleeping, too much caffeine could be your problem.

I recently met a hotel manager, Carlos, who told me he drinks about six cups of coffee throughout the day, stopping at 4 p.m. Initially, he had a hard time believing that this caffeine could be the cause of his insomnia, but he does now. Even if we assume that Carlos' cups of coffee contained just 100 mg, and using the average four-hour half-life, there's likely to still be more than 100 mg floating in his bloodstream when he turns out the light at night. Beware: long after you feel the effects of caffeine, it may still be lurking in your bloodstream.

Cutting Back on Caffeine

If you want to cut back on caffeine, realize that a tolerance for caffeine can develop in a short period of time. Caffeine also has withdrawal symptoms that usually kick in about twelve hours after drinking the last cup, so it's no wonder that caffeine drinkers wake up in the morning with a strong need for more caffeine. If you abruptly cut out the caffeine, you're likely to experience fatigue and fuzzy-headed thinking, followed by a wicked headache for a few days, but the fatigue can last as long as nine days. When reducing caffeine, it's best to make incremental changes such as stopping drinking a few hours earlier in the day or mixing your usual cup with increasing amounts of decaffeinated coffee over the course of several weeks.

Caffeine Content

(Averaged from multiple sources, to nearest 5 mg)

Generic Coffee	Caffeine (mg)
Decaf, 8 fl oz	5–15
Decaf espresso, 1 fl oz	5–10
Espresso, 1 fl oz	50–75
Instant coffee, 8 fl oz	50–150
Mocha, latte, cappuccino, 8 fl oz	65–175
Coffee, 8 fl oz	75–200

Branded Coffee	
McDonald's, large, 16 fl oz	135
Dunkin' Donuts, medium, 14 fl oz	180
Panera, 16.8 fl oz	190
Frozen Mocha, 16.5 fl oz	265
Starbucks, tall, 12 fl oz	260
Grande 16 fl oz	330
Venti, 20 fl oz	415
Iced Coffee, grande 16 fl oz	165
Espresso Frappuccino, venti, 24 fl oz	185

Generic Tea (ranges based on 1–5 minutes brewing)

Brewed, 8 fl oz	
Decaffeinated and Herbal	0–10
White	15
Green	20–60
Oolong	20–65
Black	45–75
Iced Tea, 12 fl oz	40–50

Branded Tea	
Arizona Iced Tea, green, 16 fl oz	15
Black, 16 fl oz	30
Nestea Unsweetened Iced Tea Mix, 8 fl oz, prepared	20–30
Lipton 100% Natural Lemon Iced Tea, bottle, 20 fl oz	35
Pure Leaf Iced Tea, 18.5 fl oz	60
Snapple Lemon Tea, 16 fl oz	60
Starbucks Tazo Tea, grande, 16 fl oz	

Green Tea Latte, iced or regular	80
Chai Tea Latte	95
Earl Grey, brewed or latte	115
Awake, brewed or latte, grande, 16 fl oz	135

Soft Drinks (per 12 oz)

7-Up, Fanta, Fresca, Sprite, ginger ale	0
Barq's diet root beer and most other root beer	0
Barq's Root Beer, regular	25
A&W Creme Soda	30
Coke, Coke Zero, Pepsi, Diet Pepsi, Dr. Pepper, Sunkist	35–40
Diet Coke	45
Mountain Dew, regular or diet	55

Energy Drinks

Starbucks Refreshers, 12 fl oz	50
Ocean Spray Cran-Energy, 20 fl oz	55
V-8 V-Fusion + energy, 8 fl oz	80
Red Bull, 8.4 fl oz	80
AMP Energy Boost Original, 16 fl oz	140
Monster Energy, NOS Energy Drink, Rockstar, 16 fl oz	160
Full Throttle, 16 fl oz	200
5-Hour Energy, 1.9 fl oz	210

Other Food and Beverages

Chocolate doughnut, brownie, or cake	1-15
Chocolate syrup, 2 Tbsp	2
Chocolate milk, 8 fl oz or chocolate ice cream, ½ cup	2-5
Dove Dark Chocolate Silky Smooth Promises, 5 pieces	5
Milk chocolate, 1 oz	5
Hot cocoa, 8 fl oz	15
Chocolate-coated coffee beans, 1 bean	20
Dark chocolate, 1 oz	20
Hershey's Special Dark chocolate bar, 1.5 oz	20
Starbucks hot chocolate, grande, 16 fl oz	25
Coffee or mocha ice cream, ½ cup	30

Medications

Anacin, 2 tablets (or 1 maximum strength)	65
Midol Complete, 2 caplets	120

Excedrin Migraine or Menstrual, 2 tablets	130
Excedrin Extra Strength, 2 tablets	130
NoDoz or Vivarin, 1 tablet	200

Sources: Center for Science in the Public Interest (Dec 2012), Journal of Food Science (2010), USDA National Nutrition Database for Standard Reference, product labels and websites.

4

Take Strategic Breaks

Dana is a telecom programmer analyst who has a sit down meeting with her team in San Francisco at 9:00 a.m. and a Skype session with her counterpart in India at 6:30 p.m. – which is 7:00 a.m. in New Delhi. She loves the global challenges and opportunities of her job, but it makes for a long day, so Dana's heart sinks when she feels herself hitting the wall in the middle of the afternoon.

"Of all the great ideas we've drawn from other cultures," she says, "why couldn't Americans embrace the siesta?"

Dana thinks the best she can hope for is a second wind, but I know that once she understands the physiological reason for these periodic dips in energy level (it stems from the body's internal rhythm that causes fluctuations in alertness levels), I can help her find a way to recharge and counter these energy drops. A full-on stretch-out-under-the-desk siesta isn't an option, but regular, planned recovery breaks are not only essential for optimal energy, they help us work harder and be more productive during the day.

OUR NINETY-MINUTE ALERTNESS CYCLES

More than fifty years ago, Dr. Nathaniel Kleitman, one of the researchers who connected REM sleep with dreaming, suggested that our body continually experiences ninety-minute cycles in alertness, not only during sleep (see Chapter 2), but during the day as well. During these ninety-minute cycles we experience alertness levels flowing from high to low and back to high; this 24 hour cycle is referred to as the ultradian rhythm.

While these rhythms cause extreme sleepiness during the wee hours of the night, they are also responsible for alertness flagging during the afternoon hours of 1–3 p.m. The more sleep deprived we are, the more intense we feel this afternoon fatigue. While most of us are aware when we nod off, we may not realize when we've experienced microsleep episodes (slow eye movements and brain waves typical of nighttime sleep).

Instead of living our lives in a slow and steady pace like a marathoner to conserve energy, we are more productive if we act like a sprinter, working hard for about ninety minutes and then taking a break. Taking short, regular breaks every ninety minutes or so is not only beneficial, it is essential to REBOOT energy, performance, and productivity.

REBOOT WITH RECOVERY BREAKS

Our bodies and brains get fatigued after working for long periods of time, especially when the work is repetitive or difficult. Taking a break is helpful on a number of levels:

- **Physically:** Sitting too long (see Chapter 12) is bad for our health, so we must regularly get up and move. Taking recovery breaks also prevents repetitive strain injuries to your eyes, wrists, neck, and back. Mentally exhausting activities can also impair our workouts. It's not that using your brain reduces actual muscle strength, it's that the brain perceives the exercise as harder, so we don't push ourselves as far.

- **Emotionally:** Recovery breaks improve mood, willpower, and even decision-making ability. We make so many decisions in a day that when we take our breaks matters. The decision-making process becomes less effective approaching break time and improves back to normal after the break.

- **Mentally:** Recovery breaks help us avoid making errors, keep us creative, and improve our overall mental performance. If you have ever stared at the computer screen in the grip of "writer's block" only to find that creative ideas just pop into your mind during a walk or a shower, you understand what I'm saying. While it's tempting to put your nose to the grindstone in an attempt to get the job done, remember that mental concentration works similarly to a muscle in that it becomes fatigued after sustained use and needs a rest period. This is because the brain gradually stops registering a sight, sound, or feeling that remains constant. This makes sense if you have ever experienced the deconditioning effect of a loud or annoying sound over a period of time. This is why taking short breaks throughout the day RE-BOOTS your brain to help you stay focused, attentive, and alert.

The Best Time to Take a Break

Taking a short five- to fifteen-minute break every ninety minutes has been shown to reduce fatigue, improve productivity, and reduce the risk of errors or accidents, especially when work is either demanding or monotonous. But some people work in even shorter bursts of time, needing a breather every fifteen minutes or a two-to five-minute break every thirty to forty minutes. To see what works best for you, pay attention to your productivity level and take a break when it begins to wane, rather than when it's well past due.

TO NAP OR NOT TO NAP

Naps are not just for older people. Research indicates that people of all ages and in all parts of the world nap regularly. Here's why: the longer we're awake, the sleepier we feel. Taking a planned nap (versus simply nodding off at work or at the wheel) refreshes and REBOOTS the brain circuits to improve alertness and energy level. A nap can be helpful after a normal night sleep, but it is even more beneficial to compensate for a poor night's sleep.

If you're like our globe-straddling friend Dana – always fighting mid-afternoon fatigue – you know it is more complicated than simply getting more sleep at night. Researchers compared three possible antidotes to the afternoon energy drop:

- Add an extra ninety minutes of nighttime sleep (the average person slept an additional seventy-four minutes)
- Take up to a twenty-minute nap
- Ingest 150 mg caffeine (an average cup of coffee)

More sleep, a nap, and caffeine were all effective in reducing fatigue (measured by the time it took to fall asleep in the afternoon and evening) compared to the group that changed nothing. The nap was most effective, next was caffeine, then adding more sleep. In some situations, caffeine (200 mg) plus a nap worked better in tandem than alone.

If you plan to take a short nap and then wake to a cup of coffee, do it backwards. Caffeine takes about 30 minutes to get into your system, so it's best to drink it first and follow it with a brief nap. By the time you wake up, the caffeine will be in your bloodstream!

How Long to Nap

The key to feeling refreshed is to take a short nap. While research has shown that ten minutes provides more benefits than thirty or ninety seconds, some people claim they feel rejuvenated with only seconds of sleep. A gentleman in my audience once told me that he would relax in a comfortable desk chair with a pen in his hand. When he fell asleep the pen would drop to the floor and wake him. That split second nap was enough to make him feel refreshed.

Limiting a nap to ten to twenty minutes is best because it keeps you in the lighter stages of sleep. Longer thirty- to sixty-minute naps don't provide any more alertness and will probably make you feel worse. Recall the discussion of the ninety-minute sleep cycles (see Chapter 2): the longer the nap, the greater the likelihood of falling into deep sleep. If you're sleep deprived, you will fall faster into a deep stage of sleep resulting in feeling groggy and mentally impaired when you awaken. This is called sleep inertia. While this feeling usually dissipates in ten to fifteen minutes, it can take longer. (For me, it seems to last the rest of the day.) Therefore, it's best to limit naps to ten to twenty minutes, unless you have time to complete a full ninety-minute sleep cycle.

Nap for Health

Most studies agree short naps can decrease your risk of cardio-vascular disease and loss of cognitive function during the day. One study found that habitual napping (three or more times a week) for less than thirty minutes was associated with an 84% decrease in the risk of developing Alzheimer's disease. But frequent and longer naps (forty-five minutes or longer) may negatively impact night-time sleep quality and increase the risk of heart attacks. This may be because excessive naps, long naps, and sleepiness are often indicators of poor nighttime sleep habits, sleep disorders, and psychiatric illnesses including depression, each of which is associated with an increased risk of death and disease. So keep those naps short and beneficial.

The Best Time to Nap

The best time to take a nap is when you're at your sleepiest because you'll fall asleep faster. If you're sleep deprived, that might be around noon, but otherwise the best time is around 2:00 or 3:00 in the afternoon, when your body is in that circadian slump. Short naps before 4 p.m. usually don't disrupt nighttime sleep patterns unless you have insomnia or another sleep disorder. See what works best for you.

Napping for Night-Shift Work

A nap later in the day might keep you up later at night, but that's a plus if you're working the night shift. Night shifts can be dangerous because the circadian rhythm makes unintentional sleep more likely, not only during the evening work shift but especially on the way home from work in the early morning. Taking a nap, even if it's only a light sleep, before the first night shift can help reduce the desire to sleep during the night.

Naps *during* the night shift itself may also be helpful. Nighttime naps have been tested in a number of critical situations. Critical-care nurses who napped regularly during breaks reported improved energy levels, mood, vigilance, and decision-making abilities. An oilfield service company decreased vehicle accidents by 30% by instituting a program advising drivers to take a fifteen-to twenty-five-minute nap when they got tired.

One study examined the effects of pilots taking forty-minute naps on overseas flights (while two other pilots flew the plane). The naps increased objective results of performance and alertness, quicker response time, and significantly fewer lapses in attention during the last ninety minutes of the flight, including the descent. The American Medical Association strongly recommends that regulatory agencies establish policies and procedures to ensure adequate preflight crew rest and criteria for the use of in-flight, in-cockpit napping when safe to do so during extended flights. While several large foreign airlines including British Airways, Quantas, and some

Asian carriers allow napping, not all airlines do. Another study with air traffic controllers compared a forty-minute nap with a no-nap condition. While most nappers slept for only about eighteen minutes, it resulted in improved reaction time, improved measures of alertness and performance, and reduced the likelihood of micro-sleep events (slow rolling eye movements).

REBOOT WITH NAPS

When you're in need of a REBOOT, take a brief nap using these guidelines:

- **Be sure to set a back-up alarm** if you're new to napping and are concerned that you'll fall asleep for too long.

- **Find a somewhat comfortable place** – which is easy if you're fortunate enough to work for Apple, Nike, Google, Procter & Gamble, the Huffington Post, and other companies that reported-ly offer nap rooms with recliners or a specially designed Energy Pod. Most of us have to make do lying down on the office floor, tilting our head back in a chair, or resting it on a desk. Another popular method is to go to the car and recline the seat.

- **Relax and don't be concerned about whether you fall asleep or not**. Benefits can be realized from simple relaxation. Listen-ing to nature sounds or a bubbling water fountain can also help. If you can't relax, try focusing on the rhythmic nature of your breathing. Try to slow it down by counting to four as you breathe in and counting to four as you exhale.

While not for everyone, naps are a very effective way to reboot the body when you're crashing. It may be a learned experience; regular nappers tend to fall asleep more easily and experience even more benefits than those who seldom or never nap.

REBOOT TIPS WHEN YOU CAN'T NAP

Unfortunately, most companies heavily frown on employees napping. So, when your productivity diminishes, try one of these solutions:

- **Close your eyes:** Just a minute or two helps to relieve eye strain, especially if you spend most of your time staring at the computer.

- **Take a brief mental break:** Listen to some soothing music, read a fun article, play a video game, explore on Pinterest, or just give yourself a moment to focus on your breathing or daydream.

- **Get up and move:** Stand up and do something physical. Depending on who's around, you could get up and dance, take the hoola hoop for a spin, run a few flights of stairs, or do a few simple stretches or yoga moves.

- **Shine the light:** Some studies show that using bright-light therapy (see Chapter 3) mid-afternoon might be just as effective as naps.

- **Change the scenery:** Take a walk or take your task to another room such as the cafeteria during off-hours. While taking in the sights and sounds of nature appear to be especially beneficial, walking through busy streets are not. If you can't get outside, consider looking at pictures of nature or watch a nature video. Looking at indoor plants is also relaxing.

- **Recharge with inspiration:** Get some inspiration by reading a motivational book or watching a TED talk.

- **Change the mood:** Listen to a short comedy clip for a good belly laugh. Meditation and journaling can relieve stress. Express your gratitude: take a few minutes to write a thank-you note or recommend colleagues on LinkedIn.

- **Switch tasks:** When you're stuck on a problem that needs a creative solution, switch to another task that requires less focus. The solution to the original problem may just come to you. You could organize your office files or check your email. If you work in an office at home, clean a few dishes or put in a load of laundry.

- **Ask for another perspective:** Get up and ask your colleague for some advice.

- **Take a vacation:** Vacations have been shown to spike productivity, yet many people don't take all of their allocated vacation days. Many who do take their full vacation days still feel vacation deprived — probably because they tend to regularly check their work email and voicemail.

- **Set healthy boundaries between work and home:** This could involve shutting down the phone and avoiding email over the weekend, in the evenings, or at least during the dinner hour.

- **Rehydrate:** The human body is 60% water, and dehydration affects our energy and performance. Take a break for a beverage of your choice. While caffeine helps with attention and focus, it's not a substitute for a recovery break, so enjoy it away from your desk.

- **Nourish your body:** Food is critical for energy, the ability to stay on task, manage stress, and stay emotionally balanced. So always eat your lunch and healthful snacks as needed to keep your blood glucose stable.

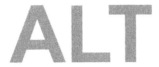

Discover an Alternate Food Pattern

"Alex and I can't face another diet," Jen tells me. "It's always the same. We starve ourselves for six weeks, and he drops fifteen pounds that don't stay off. Meanwhile, I'm lucky to drop even a few. And we're both so tired and grumpy, all we want to do is sit in front of the TV with beer and pizza."

I've got good news for her. Not a diet. It's an eating strategy designed to REBOOT energy. Weight loss (or healthy weight maintenance) is a natural side effect of an informed, energized lifestyle. We tend to forget that a calorie is a unit of measurement, and it doesn't measure fat, weight, guilt, pleasure, or sin. Calories are used to measure one thing: *energy.* So make those calories work for you!

This section of REBOOT offers an alternate food pattern to provide you with more focus, energy, and productivity. You'll learn which foods are more energizing, how much to eat, and the best time to eat, along with the importance of adequate hydration. Lastly, we'll discuss the pros and cons of stimulants such as caffeine in coffee, tea, some sodas, and energy drinks. Let's start with six simple guidelines to help you manage your energy through food and drink:

- Listen to your body talk (no, you're not crazy)

- Check your fuel gauge

- Refuel on a regular basis

- Consider the fuel mix

- Check the fluid level and energy boosters

- Eat what you love

5

Listen to Your Body Talk (No, You're Not Crazy)

Rick, a top-level Fortune 100 executive, had absolutely no problems staying sharp, focused, and energized during his hectic ten-hour workday. When he left the office, he was almost giddy with anticipation about spending the evening with his family. All that changed on the drive home when his energy level crashed. By the time he got to his front door, it wasn't just his physical energy that was waning; he was grumpy and impatient with his wife and family.

A former client of mine, Sara, told me that her hunger was uncontrollable and worried that there might be something psychologically wrong with her. After work, she picked up her son at day care, drove home, and then went into the kitchen to start dinner. As soon as she opened the pantry, though, she said she got "lost," eating everything in sight.

While the complaints of these two individuals couldn't be more different, the cause is the same. Sara ate very little during the day, saying she wasn't hungry for breakfast and didn't have time for lunch. Finally, just before dinnertime, her body screamed "Enough!" and demanded the fuel it was deprived of all day, leading to the raid on the pantry. Rick didn't fuel himself enough during the day either, relying instead on stress and caffeine to keep him going. While stress and caffeine precipitate stimulating effects, they don't fuel the body.

We sometimes forget that our bodies run on food. In fact, if you look up the word "calorie" in the dictionary, you'll find it's a measure of energy. But having energy isn't just about eating the right number of calories per day; it's about eating the *right* type of calories, at the *right* time, in the *right* quantity.

When you fuel your body in alignment with how you expend this fuel, you'll be energized, focused, productive, and emotionally balanced. In addition, your weight normalizes and is easier to maintain because eating this way controls food cravings and overeating. If you're eating enough calories throughout the day, you should feel energized. If you're feeling sluggish at any time during the day, let's find out why.

FROM BOLERO TO BALANCED

Even if you're not into classical music, chances are you've heard of Ravel's "Bolero," which was made popular with the 1979 romantic comedy "10" starring Dudley Moore and Bo Derek. It's a 15-minute piece that starts off quietly and then builds in a continuous crescendo to a thunderous intensity. Like Rick and Sara, that's how many of us eat. We start off slowly with little or no breakfast and with large gaps of time between fueling. As the day continues, we start eating more food at each sitting and more often, finishing the day with our largest meal, usually close to bedtime. But, that's not how our body needs or uses fuel.

THE BODY'S NEED FOR FUEL

The body burns calories on a steady 24/7 basis, even when we're asleep, and it uses a lot more than you realize. All our cells and organs burn fuel nonstop: the heart pumps blood, the lungs inflate with oxygen to breathe, the liver and kidney detoxify and cleanse, and the brain uses fuel to coordinate all of it. The body also uses some calories to repair itself and produce new red blood cells, hormones, enzymes, and antibodies to keep us healthy. While we may look the same from day to day, we're not. Every one of our cells (muscles, bone, skin, and more) breaks down on a regular basis and needs to be replaced. So, while we often think of ourselves as doing *nothing* when we sleep, the body is actively burning plenty of calories.

Calculating the Resting Metabolic Rate

Our resting metabolic rate (the calories needed just to stay alive) represents about 60–75% of our total calorie need.

To estimate your resting metabolic rate, use this simple one-step formula: multiply your weight by:

- 10 if you're overweight
- 11 if you're a normal-weight female
- 12 if you're a normal-weight man

So, the resting metabolic rate of a 150-pound overweight woman would be 1500 calories (150 × 10). A normal-weight active 200-pound man has a resting metabolic rate of about 2400 calories (200 × 12). Even when you want to lose weight, never eat fewer than this number of calories. Eating too few calories only lowers your metabolism, making it more difficult to continue to lose weight and keep it off.

Total Calorie Needs

Of course, because you probably don't have the luxury of spending all day in bed, let's calculate how many calories you need based on a normal day of activity. To do this, multiply your resting metabolic rate (calculated above) by one of the following factors based on your overall activity level:

- 1.2 for sedentary (sit most of the day and get little physical activity)
- 1.4 for light (such as teachers who spend most of the day on their feet or those who walk leisurely 1-3 times a week)
- 1.5 for moderately active (such as food servers who walk briskly every day or those who participate in exercise 3-5 times a week)
- 1.7 for very active (such as bike messengers or those who participate in 60 minutes of intense exercise or sports nearly every day)
- 2.0 for extremely active (those who participate in hours of exercise a day)

For example, the 150-pound woman with a light activity level would require about 2100 calories (1500 × 1.4) to maintain her weight. A 200-pound very active man would need closer to 4080 calories (2400 × 1.7). Keep in mind that these are estimates. Two people of the same size and activity level may burn calories differently for many reasons. Those with more muscle mass burn more calories, and younger people burn more calories than older individuals. Total calorie needs may also be greater in individuals who stand more than sit or those who fidget more.

Weight Loss

The numbers above are for weight *maintenance*. To lose weight you'll want to eat fewer calories than your body needs. To start losing a pound a week you can choose to eat 500 calories per day fewer than your body needs, bump up your movement to burn an extra 500 calories, or make a 250 calorie change in *both* what you eat *and* how you move. Realize that as you lose weight, you need fewer calories to maintain that weight so you'll need to adjust these numbers periodically. Appendix D offers additional tips to successfully lose weight and keep it off.

WHEN TO EAT: IT'S ALL IN THE TIMING

In order to REBOOT your energy, you need to eat in alignment with your body's needs. We do this naturally when we are babies by eating small amounts on a regular basis throughout the day. But over the years we gravitate further and further from this healthy pattern. No, I'm not suggesting that we set the alarm to wake up in the middle of the night to eat, but we do need to eat fairly evenly throughout our waking hours. Unless you're very active, you need to eat roughly one-third of your calories in the morning, one-third in the afternoon, and one-third in the evening.

There's generally no need to *count* calories, but if you want to stay energized, it helps to be more *conscious* of calories because calories are a measurement of energy. For example, if you need 2000 calories a day, it becomes clear that eating only a 200-calorie bowl of cereal and skim milk for breakfast isn't nearly enough to fuel your body throughout the morning, even if your goal is to lose weight. On the other hand, eating a 1500-calorie lunch is too much fuel and will leave you feeling sleepy mid-afternoon.

When Rick and Sara more closely adapted their day's intake to their body's needs by eating more during the day, they discovered their energy level increased during the day and their evening eating naturally fell more into alignment with their actual calorie needs. For example, Sara found out she needed around 1800 calories a day. When she started eating 600 calories in the morning and 600 calories in the afternoon, she wasn't as hungry when she came home from work. A few months later, feeling more energized, she started working out in the morning and added even more calories to her morning meal.

The 50/50 Fat-Glucose Fuel Mix

When I suggest this more balanced approach to fuel their body, people frequently respond, "But, I'm not hungry during the day. Besides, I'd rather eat less during the day so I can burn off more fat." Unfortunately, the body doesn't work that way. It's no coincidence that both breakfast skipping and weight have increased over the past 30 years. Not only can we not thrive by burning solely body fat as fuel, we won't even survive. While many factors can influence the actual moment-to-moment ratio, the body burns an average of 50% fat and 50% glucose as fuel. So, if you overeat at dinner (and increase your body fat), you're unlikely to burn off all that extra fat by skipping breakfast the next day. Worse yet, you'll be breaking down muscle mass. Here's why:

While an adult brain weighs in at just 2% of total body weight, this *motherboard* requires a total of 500 calories of glucose delivered on a consistent basis throughout the day. An additional 200 calories of glucose is needed for other non-flex-fuel parts (body parts that rely on glucose alone as fuel), including nerves, bone marrow, and the red blood cells that carry oxygen to and carbon dioxide away from every cell. In total, we need a minimum of 700 calories of glucose every day.

This glucose comes from carbohydrates (carbs): everything from bread, cereal, beans, fruits, milk, and even cookies. If we don't eat enough carbohydrates, or if we skip a meal entirely, the body has to get glucose from another source to fuel the brain and red blood cells. Unfortunately, the body has very limited stores of glucose, and fat cannot be converted into glucose. There's barely 20 calories of glucose floating in the blood stream (less than you'd find in a small piece of hard candy). That's because the bloodstream is a transportation system, not a storage depot. Even when full to capacity, liver glycogen stores contain just 400 calories, barely adequate to fuel the brain and red blood cells through the night. By morning, the body's only option is to convert muscle protein into glucose, unless it's refueled (with breakfast)

So, if you overeat at dinner and then skip breakfast, you will definitely burn some of that excess body fat as fuel. Our heart, liver, and resting muscles love to burn fat as a fuel. But, to meet the mandatory glucose requirement, the body will need to break down lean muscle mass as well. The longer you go without eating, the more muscle protein you'll need to burn. So next time you skip a meal, visualize PacMan® chewing up the muscles you worked so hard to build at the gym.

How to Burn More Fat

Perhaps you've seen headlines about how to burn more fat. Some suggest skipping breakfast, exercising in the morning before breakfast, or eating fewer carbs to burn more fat. Is there any truth behind these headlines? Yes, some. If you skip breakfast your body has no choice but to burn more fat. And, if you eat fewer carbs, the body can't make glucose, so of course you'll be burning more fat as a fuel. The same thing happens when you exercise *before* eating breakfast.

But don't confuse "burning more *fat*" with burning more *body fat*. It just means that instead of a 50/50 glucose:fat burn ratio, it might burn 40/60. The bottom line is that you're not burning more calories than usual (a basic requirement if you want to lose weight); you're just changing where the fuel is coming from. The brain and red blood cells continue to have a constant need for glucose. If you don't eat breakfast, don't eat carbs, or exercise before breakfast, the body will require the breakdown of protein to change into glucose. And that's not good. Not only does muscle mass help us look trim, it's muscle protein that keeps up your metabolism. The more we have, the higher our metabolic rate – which means we burn more calories! This is one of the reasons why men typically can eat more calories than women: they have more muscle mass.

The Call of the Siren

People often ask me how to control their appetite so they don't eat as much in the evening. What they are looking for are ways to increase their *willpower* because they think controlling their evening appetite will solve their weight problem. But, they have it backwards. Evening cravings aren't the problem; they are merely the result of not feeding the body enough during the day. When you skip or skimp on a meal, hunger eventually catches up with you, and you'll end up eating more than your body needs. It could be a few hours after the skipped meal or not until many hours later, but eventually, you'll feel an uncontrollable, irresistible attraction to food, like the calling of a siren.

In Greek mythology, sirens were half-woman, half-bird creatures that lured sailors to their death with their beautiful voices. Sometimes vending machines, descriptions of food on a menu, or whatever is in the kitchen can lure us like a siren to overeat, too. Brian Wansink, Ph.D., director of the Cornell Food and Brand Lab, investigated what people buy when they grocery shop in a hungry state. Turns out, shopping hungry didn't translate into buying more food, but it did result in buying more *high-calorie* foods. One reason for this choice might have to do with lower than normal blood glucose levels. Going too long without adequate food can drop blood glucose levels below normal (70–99 mg/dL). Even brief declines in blood glucose of about 6% seem to increase hunger and the desire to eat, even when glucose is in the normal range.

Another reason is related to the brain's reward center. In one study, researchers performed brain scans on healthy, nonobese individuals on two different mornings just before the noon hour. One time they were instructed to eat the breakfast of their choice until they were full. Another time they were instructed to skip breakfast. When shown pictures of food, the brains of the breakfast skippers lit up, revealing activity in the area of the brain that's linked to the reward value and pleasantness of food. The response was stronger with high-calorie food. The response wasn't as strong in those who ate breakfast.

So stop blaming and shaming yourself. It's almost impossible to rely on mental willpower to avoid eating high-calorie foods because extreme hunger is physiological. The brain needs a steady flow of blood glucose to keep the body alive. If you eat early in the day when your body needs the fuel, you will possess the ability to control those cravings later in the day. Sure, you'll still know where to find the high-calorie foods, but they won't tempt you like a mystical siren.

JUMP START YOUR DAY WITH BREAKFAST

Staying at a B&B on the outskirts of Paris, Andrew and Libby were treated to a typical French *petit dejeuner* every morning: an attractively presented spread of fruits, cheeses, flatbreads, and coffee.

"We didn't feel like we were eating a lot," says Libby, "but it was so beautiful and delicious, we felt totally satisfied."

More important: they were fortified for a long morning of sightseeing and tourist tromping. Back home in Indianapolis, Libby started wondering if their grab-and-go toast and coffee might be responsible for the mid-day energy slump they both experienced.

Adele Davis, a prominent and popular nutrition author in the 1960s, gave this great advice: "Eat breakfast like a king, lunch like a prince, and dinner like a pauper." Unfortunately, that's not how most of eat. If breakfast is eaten at all, it often tends to be just a snack or a beverage, and it is usually rushed like it's not an important meal.

Benefits of Eating Breakfast: Better Performance, Health, and Weight

This first meal of the day breaks your nightly fast. Breakfast provides the brain and red blood cells with much-needed glucose, stops the cannibalization of muscle mass, and replenishes glycogen stores that the body uses for fuel between meals. This process keeps the energy level and the resting metabolic rate high. Skip breakfast, and your body starts using lean muscle mass to meet its glucose needs.

There's quite a lot of research being done regarding the benefits of breakfast on improved academic performance, behavioral problems, and mood. Breakfast eaters showed quicker responses, made fewer errors on attention tasks, and improved short-term and long-term memory.

In addition, breakfast improves all aspects of mood ranging from alertness to contentment, especially when performing difficult tasks. A large study with more than 800 nurses found that those who ate breakfast more frequently reported lower stress and fewer errors at work. These regular breakfast eaters were also half as likely to have an accident or minor injury at work compared with those who eat it more irregularly.

Breakfast eaters adopted other healthy eating habits, too. Breakfast eaters tended to eat more fruits and vegetables, while breakfast skippers had higher intakes of high-fat snacks and sugary drinks. In the Health Professionals Follow-Up Study of more than 50,000 male health professionals who consumed breakfast were less likely to smoke, had lower intakes of alcohol and fat, and had higher intakes of fiber and whole grains. Breakfasts high in whole grains and fiber help reduce insulin resistance, an indicator of impending diabetes.

Eating breakfast is also linked to a reduced risk of obesity, type 2 diabetes, and heart disease. A 2012 study followed 5000 men *without* diabetes for 18 years and found that those who ate breakfast every day are 43% less likely to become obese, 34% less likely to develop type 2 diabetes, and 40% less likely to gain fat around their abdominal area (a risk factor for diabetes and heart disease) than those who ate breakfast three or fewer times a week.

If you are one of the many who put off that first meal of the day because of concerns about weight gain, believing that breakfast sets you up for constant hunger and continual nibbling all day long, or if you try to "save" calories by skipping breakfast altogether, it's time to rethink your logic about breakfast because we now know that the exact opposite holds true. Breakfast eaters tend to be leaner. The National Weight Control Registry, a database of people who have lost at least thirty pounds and kept it off for at least one year, found that eating breakfast on a regular basis was nearly twice as high in this group of successful weight-loss maintainers than the average population.

While most of us eat breakfast as kids, the trend of skipping breakfast increases as we age, along with the tendency to gain weight. Yes, breakfast skippers gained more weight than those who eat breakfast. The Health Professionals Follow-Up Study found a difference of about 12 pounds weight gain over the 10-year follow-up period. It doesn't sound like much until you consider the fact that the average American adult gains about a pound a year.

Interestingly, other controlled studies found that people who eat breakfast end up consuming *more* calories throughout the day than those who skip it, yet they are still leaner. Two reasons have been suggested for this. First, fueling the body when it needs it encourages more movement, and studies back this up by showing that breakfast eaters are more physically active. Second, breakfast helps prevent overeating during the rest of the day. Dr. Wansink recruited more than 100 people who were randomly assigned to two groups. Half were instructed not to eat for 18 hours prior to a lunchtime study. When they arrived, they were presented with a lunch buffet. Those who skipped breakfast went straight for the starchy foods and ate approximately 50% more calories of it than the control group that was permitted to eat breakfast.

Breakfast: No Excuses

While 92% of American adults agree that breakfast is the most important meal of the day, less than half are eating it every day for a variety of reasons, none of which have any validity. Here's my rebuttal to the most common of these excuses:

- **I don't have time:** Breakfast doesn't have to take a lot of time. How long does it take to prepare a peanut butter sandwich to eat with a glass of milk and a piece of fruit? Appendix E includes plenty of quick breakfast ideas, including some from fast food restaurants that take less time to order than a gourmet cup of coffee.

- **I hate breakfast foods:** There's no rational reason to limit yourself to traditional breakfast foods in the morning, just eat what you like.

- **I am not hungry:** Generally speaking, it's good advice to only eat when you're hungry, but *not* when it comes to breakfast. Even if breakfast makes you nauseous (nausea can be a sign of extreme hunger), I recommend you develop a breakfast habit. Morning anorexia is common in those who consume a lot of calories in the evening. If you don't feel hungry because you've gotten yourself into a pattern of ignoring your hunger all day and then stuffing yourself from dinner until bedtime, it's time to reconsider eating breakfast. Giving yourself permission to consume the calories you need to fuel your body during the day will help overcome nighttime eating and the weight gain that accompanies it. Initially, you might have to make yourself eat in the morning, so start with something small like a banana, whole grain toast with peanut butter, or a cup of yogurt – whatever appeals to you. If you really can't stomach something as soon as you get up, eat as early as you are able. Do not wait until lunchtime. Once you get in the habit of eating breakfast, you'll find yourself waking up hungry and craving breakfast. Don't laugh: it works!

- **Breakfast makes me hungry:** If you skip breakfast because eating early leads to hunger around 10 a.m., realize that breakfast is *supposed* to be followed by hunger a few hours later. It's normal and healthy. Any meal, even a large one, only provides about four hours of fuel. Instead of interpreting hunger as bad, start thinking of hunger as a sign that your metabolism is picking up and it's time to refuel.

- **Breakfast makes me sleepy and fuzzy headed:** It isn't breakfast, per se, that causes this feeling, but rather when, how much, and what you eat at breakfast. The longer you put off eating, the more likely you'll eat at the next meal, and it's eating a large meal that makes you sleepy.

Whatever your excuse to skip breakfast, and no matter how true your excuses might feel, the solution is not to put off eating. The longer you go without eating, the more likely you will experience negative effects such as fatigue, headache, and out-of-control cravings. Eating shortly after you wake up will REBOOT your energy and focus, preserve lean muscle mass, keep your weight down, and give you the energy you need to get through the day. So, the next time your energy drops, your mood gets negative, or you get overly hungry at 3 or 5 or 7 p.m., don't immediately start thinking you're crazy or your eating is out of control. Your body just may be telling you it's time to eat.

6

Check Your Fuel Gauge

Growing up in a family of nine kids (each just a year or two apart) meant that there were often three or four teenage drivers at home, especially during the summer months. My dad, raised in a family of mechanics, had an inexpensive solution to get us the cars we needed. He bought nonworking Volkswagen Bugs for next to nothing, replaced the nonworking parts with working ones from other Bugs to end up with a few (mostly) driving cars. One of these cars looked like Dolly Parton's "Coat of Many Colors" because it was made up of body parts from different colored cars. That wasn't so bad, except we had to enter and exit from the passenger side because the driver's side door didn't work. Another car lacked heat, so we had to wrap ourselves in a quilt when we drove it during the New York winters. Still another one of the Bugs didn't have a functioning fuel gauge, so it was critical to review the mileage of the last fill-up recorded in the small notebook tucked in the glove compartment before driving off. Failure to do this was a sure way to get stranded, trust me!

Many of you reading this are no different from this last car in regard to your internal fuel gauge. As babies, we are naturally tuned in with our fuel needs: crying when hungry and clenching our jaw shut when we've had enough. Unfortunately, as we got older, our fueling needs were overridden by our schedules and cravings. With two-thirds of the population overweight (or obese) and dragging through the day, it's obvious that many people have a nonfunctioning internal fuel gauge. We've gotten away from thinking of food as fuel. Instead, we eat out of habit, convenience, sheer pleasure, and sometimes even entertainment.

REGULATING GLUCOSE

Like a car, the body needs to always have a steady flow of fuel. It cannot run on empty. As mentioned in the previous chapter, we burn roughly 50% fat and 50% glucose as fuel throughout the day. We've got plenty of body fat to burn; a lean 154-pound man has about 135,000 calories of fat stores, but glucose stores are limited. The 400 calories of glucose stored in the liver would meet glucose needs for 12 hours (or overnight) before needing a refill. When we run out of fuel, we run out of energy.

Eating on a regular basis REBOOTs energy because it provides a steady stream of glucose. According to the American Diabetes Association, normal fasting glucose levels are within a very narrow range of 70-99 mg/dL. Both high (hyperglycemia, as is experienced in diabetes) and low (hypoglycemia) glucose levels can be life threatening and, at the very least, are associated with poor health. And both high and low glucose levels can negatively affect our focus, mood, willpower, and energy level.

Understanding how the body balances blood glucose will help you realize why eating on a regular basis is so important and how often to do so. Ideally, the body works continuously to keep plasma glucose levels within a normal range through the action of two hormones that work in a reciprocal relationship: insulin and glucagon. Insulin lowers blood glucose, and glucagon raises it.

Going Down

Most of us have gotten the message that we need to eat X number of calories *a day*, or we'll put on weight. But, that's just a small part of the REBOOT solution for boosting energy. A meal of any size takes just three to five hours to be fully digested and absorbed into the bloodstream. If we eat more than we need for *any moment in time*, we'll not only put on body fat, we will zap our energy, and here's why:

While a meal contains carbohydrate, protein, and fat, it's the carbohydrates that enter the bloodstream first, mostly in the form of glucose. This increased blood glucose level prompts the pancreas to secrete insulin, which is required to escort the glucose into the cells that need it. Due to this large influx of glucose, the body responds by switching from a 50/50 mix of fat and glucose to a fuel blend that's mostly glucose, but only for two hours following a meal.

Within those two hours, the glucose from the meal has either been used or stored, and blood glucose levels return to the normal range. This is true even after a very large meal. Remember this two-hour rule. Getting blood glucose back to the normal range in two-hours is critical for health and optimal performance. Glucose doesn't just float around the bloodstream until it's needed (remember, high blood glucose is indicative of diabetes). The body *has* to put the extra glucose calories somewhere, and there are just two storage options: glycogen (stored glucose) and fat. The liver can hold at most 400 calories of glucose, while muscles can store another 500–600 calories (though trained athletes often have a larger capacity).

Once glycogen reserves have been replenished (though keep in mind, they rarely are ever "empty" in the first place), all the remaining calories go into fat stores. That's why it's important to consider not just how many calories you eat *in a day*, but also how many calories you eat *at one time*. Larger meals (with more calories than you need for those few hours) will increase your fat stores and leave you feeling sluggish and sleepy.

Going Up

About two hours after you eat, all the carbohydrates from that meal have been used for fuel or socked away into glycogen or fat stores. This returns blood glucose levels back to normal. But as the brain and red blood cells continue to draw glucose from the blood for fuel, glucose levels begin to fall. If plasma glucose ever got too low, you could black out or even die, but this is unlikely to happen because a healthy body has systems in place to bring plasma glucose levels back up to a normal level. As soon as glucose drops even slightly below normal, the pancreas produces the hormone glucagon, which helps the body access glucose from body stores. First, it draws from the limited amount of liver glycogen. Unfortunately, it can't draw from the glycogen in muscles (it's only available as a fuel for the specific muscle it's stored in). For example, when running, your muscles use the glycogen in your leg muscles as fuel; swimming uses the glycogen stored in your arms and legs. Muscle glycogen cannot leave the muscles to fuel the brain.

Not knowing when your next meal will be, and realizing that 400 calories of liver glycogen won't last long, the body immediately starts turning protein into glucose to spare this glycogen. It burns only a small amount of protein at first, but as amounts of glycogen decrease the percent of protein increases. This protein may come from what you just ate or, sadly, from your muscles. Now you understand why it's important to always eat some carbohydrates at each meal (we'll discuss exactly how much in Chapter 8). Carbs fuel all our glucose needs for the first two hours after a meal, while liver glycogen (stored glucose) carries us through to the next meal. If you don't eat sufficient carbs, your body uses protein for fuel, which means it's not available for rebuilding the body.

THE ROLLER-COASTER EFFECT

Roller coasters are known for their climbs and their falls; the higher they climb, the faster they fall. The same thing is true for blood glucose levels. Shortly after eating, carbohydrates are digested and absorbed as glucose molecules, causing blood glucose to rise about 50% above normal fasting levels as the glucose travels through the bloodstream to the cells that need it. Just like a roller coaster's ups and downs, small meals result in smaller rises and falls in blood glucose levels, while larger meals result in bigger ones.

These rises and falls last, at most, two hours because a normal pancreas will supply enough insulin to escort the glucose where it needs to go to bring the levels back to normal within two hours (remember the two-hour rule). For the next couple of hours, the blood glucose holds fairly stable through the opposing action of insulin and glucagon until the body runs out of fuel and needs more food.

For peak performance and optimal energy, we have to be cognizant and respectful of this fuel requirement. Unfortunately, instead of fueling our bodies at the time we need the fuel, most of us go through periods of underfeeding when we skip or skimp at breakfast and possibly lunch, and then overindulge from dinner to bedtime. While a sharp rise and fall on a roller coaster may thrill you, this destructive pattern of over fueling followed by under fueling not only zaps energy, it affects mood, attention span, body composition, and productivity.

Over Fueling: Why Big Meals Don't Fuel You Longer, They Just Make You Fatter

A normal-sized meal fuels the body for three or four hours. A very large meal, and I don't care how big it is, will only provide fuel for five hours at most. At that point, the meal has been completely processed by the gastrointestinal tract and absorbed into the rest of the body. The body has used some of those nutrients for fuel and some to do repairs. Any nutrients over and above what's needed at that particular moment in time has to go somewhere, and it's not into bulging muscles (don't you wish). Excess calories don't float around in the blood stream until needed (remember high blood glucose is indicative of diabetes). Sure, some carbs might be used to top off glycogen stores, but the glycogen storage tank is small. Excess calories go straight to the fat cells. It doesn't matter whether these calories are from carbohydrates, protein, or fat: all excess calories turn to fat.

So, if you need only 600 calories at your evening meal but decide to go out for a 1500-calorie dinner (it's easy to eat that much in just one entrée, even without drinks or dessert), you'll be filling out some fat cells. A big meal doesn't provide you with more energy; it just makes you fatter.

Something else to consider is that while a large meal has the ability to provide for about five hours of fuel, you might feel that it's even less. Here's why:

The body has a specific calorie need to keep itself alive, let's say it's 1800 calories a day. So, if you eat three times a day, you're likely to eat about 600 calories per sitting. If you eat just two meals, it might be closer to 900 calories per sitting. But, if you eat just once a day, you'll be eating the 1800 calories in that one sitting. Remember the roller-coaster effect; when you eat just one or two meals a day the meals will likely be larger and blood glucose rises higher than if you ate three smaller meals. The higher the blood glucose rises, the more insulin is released, and the faster it tends to fall. And, when it does fall, it's likely to fall too low, too fast, leaving you feeling hungry, tired, and weak in just 2–3 hours, even though you ate enough calories for many more hours. This is called reactive hypoglycemia.

This should make it clear why a large meal does not make you feel energized or even fill you up longer. In fact, eating a large meal will actually make you *less full* and more tired than eating a smaller meal. The key is to never eat so much that you put your body on this roller-coaster ride resulting in feeling exhausted, irritable, and hungry.

Under Fueling: Goodbye Lean Muscle Mass

Years ago a 22 year-old woman, Celine, came to see me complaining of two things: exhaustion (her doctor had ruled out any medical causes) and cellulite. At first, I had a hard time believing that this woman, who claimed to exercise more than an hour a day (a full hour of aerobics, plus weights), could really have much of a problem with cellulite, until she showed me. Even though she was within an ideal weight range, her legs were covered with what resembled bumpy cottage cheese from butt to knee. This was clearly not normal, and I soon found out what was causing it.

I asked her what and when she ate. If she didn't skip breakfast, she had something light like a banana. Lunch was often just a green salad with fat-free dressing or an apple. She hit the gym right after work, drove home, prepared dinner, and ate a large healthy dinner (meat, carbs, and veggies) late in the evening, often with a glass of wine, followed by a snack or dessert even later. My nutritional analysis revealed that she was eating the appropriate amount of calories, proteins, carbs, and fat per day. So how could she be eating the right number of calories to maintain an ideal weight, plus the right amount of protein and doing the right amount of exercise to build muscle mass, yet have little muscle tone?

The answer to this conundrum was in the timing of her meals. Clearly she was eating enough protein to build strong muscles and working out on a regular basis. But, our bodies can use only a small amount of protein at any one time (more about this in Chapter 8). Although her evening meal contained her entire daily need for protein, her body used only a small amount of it to build muscle. Most was used to replace more important proteins such as insulin, hemoglobin in the red blood cells, and more.

And while Celine was eating the right number of calories, she consumed nearly all of them in one four-hour time period late in the day. Let's examine how those calories were being used. Her large evening meal provided adequate amounts of carbohydrates to fuel the glucose needs for the first two hours after the meal and refilled her glycogen stores. Unfortunately, because she ate too many calories for that moment in time, she also increased fat stores. While Celine slept, her body used fuel in a 50/50 glucose-fat ratio. Early in the night, that fat need came from the dinner meal, but about 4–5 hours after dinner, the body got the fat from her fat stores. Now, to meet her glucose needs, Celine burned liver glycogen with a small continually increasing amount of protein. By the time she woke up in the morning, most of her liver glycogen was gone. Therefore, most of her glucose needs were being met with protein. As the day wore on, she skimped on breakfast and lunch, requiring her body to burn more and more muscle protein to meet the glucose requirement of her brain and red blood cells.

This cyclical storage of fat from the evening meal along with burning of protein during the day resulted in Celine's increasingly fatter body composition, even with exercise. This isn't good because muscles are the calorie-burning powerhouse of the body. Less muscle mass means fewer calories burned. This is why smaller, more frequent meals help improve energy and body composition.

GETTING BACK IN TOUCH WITH YOUR HUNGER AND FULLNESS

I clearly remember the day I picked my young daughter up from daycare and put her in her car seat. She was hungry so I handed her a graham cracker square. A few minutes later, as I was driving home, she told me she'd had enough and handed me back this tiny piece, no bigger than a quarter. I almost drove off the road as I pondered how many of us adults are *that* in-tuned with our own hunger and fullness. How many of us would, even if we felt full at that moment, put down that last quarter-sized piece of cookie and say, "I've had enough"? I'm guessing most of us would simply pop that piece into our mouth.

While, in the previous chapter, I provided simple calculations to *estimate* your calorie needs as a guide for planning how much to eat throughout the day, realize that this needs be adjusted to meet your *actual* needs. So, start by planning for about one-third of your total calories during each third of the day: morning, afternoon, and evening – then modify it according to your hunger (which will fluctuate according to your activity level) throughout the day and from day-to-day. Below are some guidelines to help you stay energized while keeping your weight down (Appendix D offers additional tips).

Align Your Eating with Movement

Marissa experienced headaches and overwhelming fatigue a few days a week, and when her doctor found nothing medically wrong with her, she came to see me. Marissa was very regimented about not only eating frequently throughout the day, but also eating the same amount every day, whether she exercised or not.

None of us burn the exact same amount of calories every day, which is why it's acceptable to use estimated calorie needs as a *guide* for fuel, but we must also listen to our body for a more accurate assessment of our fuel needs. Marissa's headaches and fatigue were signs of hypoglycemia, her body's way of saying, "more, please." Once she upped her calories to match her fitness regimen, her energy came back and the headaches disappeared. For those of you worried that eating more puts on excess weight, keep in mind that if you eat more when your body needs the fuel, you're likely to feel more energized now and eat less later.

One study compared nonobese healthy women who reported symptoms of reactive hypoglycemia more than once a week with a control group who did not have symptoms. Mean blood glucose levels after the meal were significantly lower in women who complained of hypoglycemia: 84 mg/dL versus 91 for the controls. While blood glucose levels after meals did not drop below 70 mg/dL, the women with reactive hypoglycemia reported symptoms about two and a half hours after eating with an average finger prick blood glucose of 75 mg/dL. Interestingly, on those days when the women reported symptoms, they were more physically active than the controls. Therefore, it's important to match your eating to your activity level; more active days require more fuel.

Listen to Your Hunger

If your energy level needs a REBOOT, start listening more closely to your body. When you feel weak and your stomach starts to growl, feed it. Hunger is a sign that the blood glucose is dropping and you need to refuel. Then, stop eating when you're feeling satisfied but *not full*. Using this 10-point scale, I suggest you start eating when your hunger gauge gets to a 3 or 4 and stop when you're at a 5. This will give you the right amount of fuel to maintain your energy level for the next few hours.

10: Thanksgiving stuffed, feeling sick to your stomach
9: Stuffed and uncomfortable
8: Beginning to get uncomfortable, it's starting to hurt
7: Ate too much
6: More than just satisfied
5: Feeling just fine, not hungry or full
4: Starting to feel hunger
3: Clearly hungry, the urge to eat is strong
2: Very hungry, you want to eat anything that's around
1: So hungry you feel "starved to death"
0: You no longer feel hungry

I realize that there's not much of a variance between levels, but it's critical to avoid extremes. If you allow yourself to get too hungry (number 1 or 2), chances are, you'll end up overeating. As I mentioned earlier, functional imaging techniques of the brain demonstrate that being overly hungry increases the appeal of food, making it harder to resist. While many diet books suggest riding the wave or waiting until the craving disappears (a number 0), realize that you've shut off your body's ability to communicate with you about hunger. You shouldn't ignore your hunger for two reasons:

First, if you don't feed yourself when you're hungry, eventually that hunger will come back with a vengeance (recall the Call of the Siren) because the body is always looking out for you. It doesn't want you to starve to death.

Two, when you stop feeling hunger, your body has given up on you to fuel the brain, and it reaches into body stores to get the blood glucose back to the normal range. This requires breaking down both liver glycogen (if there's any left) and lean muscle mass. The longer you go without eating, the more muscle protein you burn.

Early Eater, Late Eater

For optimal energy, it's best to eat calories spaced evenly throughout waking hours rather than during a few hours. This will help you maintain a normal weight, too. Because we tend to be even more active during the day, you might even think in terms of becoming an early eater, where you eat more calories during the early part of the day. Many observational studies have shown that earlier eaters tend to be leaner than those who eat most of their calories in the evening. In some cases, researchers found the greater the proportion of calories eaten in the morning, the lower the total daily calories consumed. This makes sense because balanced eating can help control appetite.

One study compared more than 400 people on a 20-week weight-loss program who ate the same number of calories, burned the same number of calories, and slept the same amount. The early eaters (main meal eaten before 3:00 p.m.) lost more weight than the late eaters (main meal eaten after 3:00 p.m.).

In another study involving overweight and obese women on low-calorie diets, the breakfast group ate 50% of their allowed calories at breakfast with progressively fewer calories at lunch and dinner. The dinner group ate it backwards with half their calories eaten at dinner. Again, even though they consumed the same calories, the breakfast group reported greater satiety, less hunger, and in the end lost more weight and more body fat. Remember: calories matter, but so does *when* you eat those calories. Even if weight isn't an issue, concentrating calories in the evening, rather than spreading out the calories throughout the day, can negatively affect all aspects of energy including physical energy, mood, concentration, and even productivity.

Stand Up and Lose Weight

I remember a Thanksgiving feast many years ago when my daughter said something very wise. We were sitting next to each other on a very long table filled with family and friends. One by one, as people got up from the table, they would grasp their bellies and moan, "Oh, I ate too much." My wise daughter whispered to me, "Mom, if people would just stand up half-way through their meal, they would know when they ate enough, before they ate too much." So true.

Think back to a time when you had a meal interrupted. Maybe you had to take one of your young children to the bathroom or answer the phone. Did you notice when you returned to the table that your appetite wasn't as sharp? It takes 15–20 minutes for the brain to register when it's full, and a short break is helpful to cut short the repetitive fork-to-mouth motion. Let's face it, most of us put a forkful of food in our mouth, and while we're still chewing, get the next forkful ready. If you don't want to stand up and walk away from the table halfway through your meal, at least put your fork down and rest between bites and assess your hunger score.

Discover What's Eating You

If you feel like you're always hungry, or if you're eating more than your body needs (as evidenced by weight gain), then it's time to cue into what's driving the feeling of hunger. Are you *physiologically* hungry, or are you using food to satisfy an *emotional* need? Often, we eat when we're disappointed, tired, stressed, angry, worried, sad, bored, or lonely, instead of looking for a healthier option to manage our emotions.

If this describes you, start keeping a log of when you eat, what you eat, with whom you are eating, and your mood. You might want to use an app such as RiseUp by Recovery Warriors. While the app was designed for people recovering from an eating disorder, it is also useful for anyone trying to get a grasp on what they're feeling emotionally when they eat. After entering your information, you send yourself a PDF chart that enables you to see the patterns in what's prompting you to eat.

Eat Only When You Feel Hungry

We often eat for reasons other than hunger. Perhaps you need to munch on popcorn while at the movies. Maybe, no matter how full you feel, you just have to have dessert every evening. This habit of eating is driven by the time of day, a specific event, or even a smell. When we eat to satisfy true physiological hunger, we tend to compensate for those extra calories and eat somewhat less later on. On the other hand, eating when we're not hungry doesn't cause the same feedback on appetite, meaning we don't compensate for those extra calories at our next meal, causing us to overeat or consume more calories than we need.

Here's an interesting study from France that illustrates this point: Most children and some adults in France habitually eat a mid-afternoon "fourth meal" in response to hunger, referred to as *goûter* (prounounced gou-tay). (This is not to be confused with Taco Bell®'s FourthMeal, which is more of a midnight munchies thing.) Research indicates that because the goûter is eaten in response to hunger, goûter eaters compensate by eating fewer calories at other meals.

Researchers recruited young normal-weight men; half said they normally had three meals a day (and weren't hungry for an afternoon snack), while the other half were "habitual fourth-meal eaters." For a four-week period of time, each was asked to change their habit; those eating three meals a day *added* a goûter, while the goûter eaters *skipped* that meal. Adding a meal had no effect on weight, but that's probably because the researchers cut the calories at lunch by a third so study subjects were *physiologically* hungry for the goûter. You'll read more about this shortly, but it's important to snack only when you're hungry.

What about the usual goûter eaters who were asked to *skip* the snack? At the start of the study, it was noted that the higher the calories in the usual goûter, the lower the body fat. Skipping the goûter for traditional goûter eaters led to a higher calorie lunch and dinner, and to an *increase* in body fat. Interestingly, the higher the calories for the usual goûter, the more fat they gained when skipping the goûter.

Epidemiological studies have found that goûter eaters are more active than nongoûter eaters. And in this study, the goûter eaters reported eating more calories from the start than those who traditionally skipped the fourth meal, so there's a good chance they were also more active. Therefore, as will discuss in Chapter 7, snacking is a more appropriate way for active individuals to fuel their activity needs.

EAT BEFORE IT'S TOO LATE

When you go too long without eating, your blood glucose will eventually drop as your brain and red blood cells continue to soak up glucose for fuel. Just because normal, healthy bodies have mechanisms in place to bring the glucose back up doesn't mean you should put off eating. The list below outlines both the short- and long-term implications of ignoring the signs of hunger:

- **Your body burns more muscle mass:** If you hold off eating long enough, your hunger will eventually go away (as you hit 0 on the hunger scale). But, as the body works its magic to bring up the blood glucose, muscle mass is being cannibalized to provide this glucose. The longer you go without eating, the more protein is being used.

- **Your body always tries to make up the calories (and then some:** The human body tries to keep the status quo. Eventually, your appetite will increase, and you'll end up overeating in response to these symptoms, usually by eating higher-calorie foods.

- **Alertness and energy levels deteriorate:** Energy slumps last until blood glucose gets back up, and likely even longer than that. Hypoglycemia feels different for different people. Some report symptoms of feeling weak, dizzy, and tired long after blood glucose comes back up. Others feel shaky and jittery.

What's that Shaky, Jittery Feeling?

As blood glucose levels drop, the pancreas produces the hormone glucagon to bring it back up. Around that time, the body also produces the stress hormone adrenaline, which causes that shaky or jittery feeling. We all have different thresholds as to when adrenaline is produced. Some bodies respond to bring up blood glucose levels before this threshold is reached, so they don't get the jitters. Others are very sensitive and seem to feel shaky right away. There's also research to indicate that caffeine increases this threshold. So, while caffeine doesn't *cause* low blood glucose, drinking caffeine might make you *more susceptible* to this adrenaline release.

The Dangers of Hypoglycemia

Hypoglycemia can be dangerous for individuals being treated with certain diabetes drugs, including insulin, but there are ramifications even if you do not have diabetes. The more often you experience hypoglycemic symptoms, the more readily you will experience them again. In one study, researchers looking at healthy volunteers found that glucagon and adrenaline were secreted at higher plasma glucose concentrations after a previous hypoglycemic incident. It's almost like your body realizes that because you've ignored the warnings in the past, it will respond quicker the second time around. That means you might experience the shaky, jittery feeling even before your blood glucose gets too low. Recurrent hypoglycemia may have long-term health implications as well because it may promote insulin resistance, a risk factor for diabetes. A single hypoglycemic event promotes insulin resistance for seven to nine hours and for as long as eighteen hours after two brief episodes of hypoglycemia in individuals *without* diabetes.

Don't Put Off Eating

If you wait until you feel shaky or jittery before you eat, it's too late. That adrenaline-fueled shaky feeling is a sign your body is already in the process of bringing the glucose level back up. Even while your body is in the midst of chiseling away at your muscle mass to provide glucose for your brain, low blood glucose is causing you to crave sugars and starches to bring the blood glucose up quickly.

Because the symptoms last longer than the actual low-blood-glucose event, it's easy to continue to eat long after the blood glucose is back up. It takes about twenty minutes for the stomach to signal the brain that you've had enough, and the hungrier you feel, the faster you'll eat, and the more likely you are to overeat before your brain registers fullness. Also, it takes time for the adrenaline to leave your system. Think back to the last time you had a near car accident and your body secreted adrenaline. It took a long time for that shaky feeling to disappear, didn't it? The combination of the body working to bring up the blood glucose through body stores coupled with your eating (and possibly overeating) is likely to send your blood glucose on another high-low roller-coaster ride. No matter how hungry you are, overeating only perpetuates the roller-coaster effect of those glucose spikes.

Treating and Preventing Hypoglycemia

When you're feeling the symptoms of hypoglycemia, you need to eat a small snack as soon as possible that contains both carbohydrates and protein to stabilize your blood glucose. Good choices include a glass of nonfat milk, a six-ounce container of yogurt, a piece of fruit with an ounce of lower-fat cheese, a few crackers smeared with peanut butter, or a 100-calorie portion of a bar (Appendix H lists many other snack options).

If you're late in getting some food and still feeling bad, just eat protein such as jerky, a hard-boiled egg, cheese stick, a half cup of cottage cheese, or a couple of ounces of deli or leftover meat. The reason to focus on eating protein is that your body has already released glucose from glycogen stores or muscle protein to bring up the blood glucose, and there's no need to increase it further. The protein will help to stabilize the blood glucose.

Whichever dietary fix you take, remember to wait and relax after eating and keep in mind that it takes longer for the shakes to go away than it does for blood glucose to rise back to normal. Don't continue to eat.

When the symptoms subside, analyze why your glucose level got so low, so you can prevent it from happening again. Perhaps you went too long without eating or didn't eat enough to meet your activity needs. Rapidly falling blood glucose can also follow a very large meal or an unbalanced meal. Learn from your mistakes, pay closer attention to your hunger signals, and next time, eat a planned snack *before* your blood glucose gets out of control. One study found that it's possible to learn, within a short period of time, to read body symptoms and detect when blood glucose levels fall towards the low end of normal. You can learn to do this by paying close attention to the signals your body is sending you, so eventually fueling your body becomes more innate.

Remember, REBOOT isn't about counting calories, it is about becoming *calorie conscious*. If you don't fuel your body adequately at the time it needs calories, you'll experience negative side effects. The next two chapters discuss in detail what and when to eat to ensure you're eating the right food at the right time of the day. When you fill your tanks adequately, you end up with *right* amount of fuel at the *right* time for peak energy, performance, and body composition.

7

Refuel on a Regular Basis

Try as she might, Juanita always seemed to have a tough time around 3:00 p.m. Her eyelids drooped along with her energy level, making work difficult. Though she went searching for energy in the break room's coffee and vending machines, Juanita admitted these only gave her a quick fix followed by another slump. Eating regularly throughout the day is the remedy.

EAT AT LEAST THREE "REGULAR" MEALS A DAY

In Juanita's case, breakfast consisted only of coffee and a pastry. Although she tried to control her appetite at lunch, she always ended up eating more than she planned. While lack of sleep can increase a mid-afternoon slump, this was not Juanita's problem. No breakfast followed by a large lunch was the issue. In addition to eating breakfast, I suggested that instead of changing what she ordered for lunch, she ask for half of it to be boxed to go. Sometimes she ate these leftovers for another meal, and sometimes she just left the box on the table. The point is that eating only half the portion kept her more alert in the mid-afternoon. In addition, Juanita realized that her slumps were worse when she ate lunch late, so she made more of an effort to eat it on time (Appendix B offers a full list of how to deal with mid-afternoon energy crashes).

Unusually large lunches not only aggravate a mid-afternoon slump, they also increase errors. Eating three moderately sized meals each day matched to calorie needs (no under fueling, no over fueling) keeps your energy on an even keel. While there are some advantages to eating more often than this, eating a minimum of three moderately sized meals a day at regular intervals is critical to maintaining optimal health and energy. Here's why:

- **Better energy:** Irregular eaters who frequently send their blood glucose levels into a roller-coaster effect find themselves tired (from the after effects of adrenaline) and overweight (from subsequent overeating). Eating regularly helps stabilize blood glucose levels, resulting in increased energy.

- **More willpower:** Go too long without eating, and willpower and self-control fly out the window. There is a physical reason for this. Self-control and willpower rely on a limited resource, glucose, so both are reduced when glucose levels are low, but they improve when normal glucose levels are restored. Low levels of glucose also affect the ability to cope with stress, control negative emotions, and resist the temptation to smoke, overeat, and overdrink.

- **Strengthened memory, mood, and attention:** The brain relies upon a steady stream of glucose, so when you go too long without eating, basic functions like mood, memory, and attention begin to deteriorate. In fact, both low and high blood glucose levels affect the brain and, potentially, the ability to think rationally and recall memory.

- **Lower insulin, less risk of diabetes:** Larger meals tend to raise glucose higher than smaller meals, requiring more insulin to get back to a normal level. It makes sense that regular eaters have lower insulin levels than irregular eaters, which translates to having a lower risk for diabetes. Nearly 30,000 U.S. men in the Health Professionals Follow-Up Study were followed for sixteen years. Men who ate one to two times a day had a higher risk of type 2 diabetes compared with those who ate three times a day.

- **Lower LDL:** Concentrations of low-density lipoprotein (LDL), the so-called bad cholesterol, tend to be lower in people eating smaller, more frequent meals versus those who eat only one or two meals a day.

- **Satiety and appetite control:** One study found that people who ate once a day lost more weight and body fat than those who ate three meals a day, even though they totaled the same number of calories. But wait until you hear the rest of the story. All subjects were normal-weight individuals who were fed enough calories to maintain their weight. Those who ate once a day found it difficult to consume all the calories at one meal; hence, they ended up eating slightly fewer calories and dropped an average of three pounds during the six-month program. More importantly, these individuals never got used to the once-a-day meal and reported a significant increase in hunger and desire to eat throughout the day (though they didn't because this was a controlled study). In real life, hungry people tend to give in to their hunger and eat (and possibly overeat). Frequent eating helps with satiety (feeling full) and controls appetite, perhaps by reducing ghrelin levels, which decreases hunger. (Recall from Chapter 2 that ghrelin is the hormone that stimulates hunger.)

• **Weight Control:** Eating fewer than three meals a day leads to increases in body fat, while eating three moderately sized meals a day can prevent this. People in the National Weight Control Registry report that consistent eating was important for them to maintain their weight loss. Those who allowed themselves more flexibility on weekends and holidays had a *greater* risk of weight gain. This was confirmed by a study that compared the effects of healthy obese women who followed two phases of their normal diet for two weeks each: they ate a *regular* pattern of six meals a day and an *irregular* pattern where daily eating ranged from three to nine meals. During the two weeks they ate within a regular pattern, they ended up eating fewer calories than the two weeks they ate the irregular meal pattern.

TO SNACK OR NOT TO SNACK

The research is clear: a minimum of three meals a day is critical for energy, health, and weight maintenance. While adding snacks to the mix might offer additional benefits for some individuals under certain circumstances, it's clear that snacking isn't for everyone. Here's the scoop on what snacking can and cannot do for you.

Improved Health

Beyond what three meals a day can do, smaller, more frequent meals supplemented with snacks have been shown to further improve blood-lipid profiles (especially LDL cholesterol), reduce insulin levels, and improve insulin resistance (the way the body uses insulin). Limited studies indicate that eating smaller, more frequent meals reduced the incidence and severity of symptoms in those suffering from migraines and Meniere's disease (a chronic condition of dizziness and ringing in the ears). Because insulin levels were higher in individuals with migraines, smaller, more frequent meals may reduce insulin and, thus, migraine incidence.

Critical for Children

Regular eating (three meals a day plus snacks between meals) is especially critical in the developing child for several reasons:

- **A child's brain represents a much larger percentage of total body weight:** By age two, a child's brain is already 80% of the weight of an adult and requires a constant source of glucose for fuel. This helps explain why a child's caloric needs are much greater than would be expected by their body size; a tiny two-year-old toddler needs about half the calories as an average-size adult.

- **Children sleep more hours than adults:** This creates longer gaps between "fueling," so it's helpful to have both a bedtime snack and an early breakfast.

- **Children have smaller liver and muscle weights:** Because liver glycogen and muscle protein amounts are based on a percentage of their organ weights, this limits how much liver glycogen and muscle protein is available to burn as fuel between meals.

Therefore, children's calorie needs are high, and stores to sustain normal glucose levels are relatively low, which requires frequent eating to sustain stable glucose levels.

Appetite Control

Adding snacks to a three-meal-a-day eating pattern can help control appetite. When researchers divided the calories from one meal into several smaller meals, individuals tended to eat less at the next meal than when those same calories were eaten all at once. This also holds true for people who snack, as they tend to report significantly less hunger than those eating just three meals a day. This makes sense because a meal only lasts three to five hours (depending on its size). Eventually, you're going to run out of fuel, causing a slight dip in your blood glucose level, which makes you feel hungry. It's then that eating a small snack will REBOOT your energy, focus, and productivity.

May or May Not Help Weight Loss

The claim that eating frequent meals throughout the day helps you lose weight has been around for decades. Indeed, it works for some people, but not for everyone. Let me explain.

It all started with rat research. When rats, which typically nibble all day long, are restricted to receiving food just once or twice a day, they quickly adjust. Within a few days, they adjusted by eating more every time they were fed, so that they learned to consume their entire food allotment in the time allowed. These infrequent feedings led to a decrease in their activity and an increase in their fat stores.

At first, this led to the belief that eating more frequently is better for weight control. And initial studies in humans found that those who ate more frequently did appear to be leaner. But, if it's that simple, we'd all be thin! While snacking has increased among U.S. adults in the past 30 years, so has our weight.

While this overarching claim keeps circulating around on the Internet, we've discovered that it isn't quite true. In general, we all tend to report eating less and moving more than we actually do. Using more accurate laboratory technology, we've discovered that the heaviest people who reported eating the fewest meals were reporting intakes too low for their expected calorie needs. Once participants who reported implausible calorie intakes were excluded from the analyses, most of the studies showed that people who ate more often tended to weigh more.

What this means is that simply eating whatever you want on a frequent basis throughout the day will not magically cause you to burn more calories. Eating more often doesn't boost metabolism or make you lose weight. The weight equation is still about calories in versus calories out. If eating frequently controls your appetite so you eat less, then frequent eating will help you lose weight – not because you're eating more often, but because you are eating fewer calories. On the other hand, if snacking only invites more opportunities for you to overindulge, then more frequent eating won't help you lose weight.

Fuels an Active Lifestyle

Adults who eat more than three times a day tend to be heavier, with one exception: those who are physically active. For both men and women, the more active their lifestyle, the more often they tend to eat. This makes sense because athletic individuals require more calories than sedentary individuals, and frequent eating makes it easier to get the calories/fuel they need. Depending on the length of the activity, athletes should increase their intake of snacks and beverages before, during, and after exercise to replace glycogen stores and rebuild muscle (more in Chapter 13). The same would hold true of active people who burn more calories and, thus, need more fuel.

Lowers Body Fat and Preserves Muscle Mass

Snacking may also help athletes lower their body-fat percentage and preserve muscle mass during dieting (as long as protein levels are adequate). In one fascinating study, researchers compared how many calories elite athletes consumed with how many calories they burned on an hour-by-hour basis. Those with calorie intakes that most closely matched their expenditure had a lower body-fat percentage. This was true for both anaerobic (gymnasts) and aerobic (runners) elite athletes. In another study, athletes were divided into two groups where only one group was provided 250-calorie snacks to eat three times a day between meals. The snack group lost more fat, gained more muscle, and displayed both more anaerobic power and energy output in testing.

GUIDELINES FOR SNACKING

If you're active (or plan to be) and want to add snacks to your meal plan to increase your energy level, control your appetite, and fuel your activity, but are concerned that it may encourage you to overeat, here are some guidelines that can help you.

Consider Total Calories

Ideally, snacks should help control your appetite so you eat less at the next meal. But if eating more often just sets you up to over-indulge, then you'll defeat the purpose of snacking, not because you're eating frequently but because you're eating more calories.

There was a study of physically active men of normal weight in which half were given a chocolate snack six days a week for six months while the other half were asked to simply maintain their normal eating. At the end of the study, there was no significant difference in body weight between the groups because those given the chocolate snack compensated for the extra calories by eating less at meal or snack times. Some people can do this naturally, but for others, snacking is an invitation to overindulge, and they do not compensate for eating extra snack calories. Again, active individuals tend to be better able control calorie intake with snacking. Young people, too, seem to be better compensators than older individuals. Men are better than women (though some studies have indicated that this advantage disappears when men get older). Women have more of an issue compensating for extra snack calories, especially after menopause.

Weight also plays a role. While snacking in normal-weight individuals doesn't lead to increased weight, snacking in obese individuals does, even if they exercise. Therefore, overweight individuals may control their hunger and weight better by eating three evenly distributed meals and skipping the snacks.

Snack Only When Hungry

Hunger is a sign that the body needs more fuel. When we are able to snack according to our hunger level, we compensate by eating less at the next meal. Recall the goûter studies in Chapter 6 about the fourth-meal in France served in response to hunger. Traditional goûter eaters were hungry at snack time. Ignoring this hunger (like those who were asked to skip the goûter) leads to eating a higher calorie lunch and dinner, ultimately resulting in an increase in body fat.

In order to snack to control appetite and not pack on the pounds, you must snack only in response to hunger. When you don't feel physiologically hungry at snack time (a 3 or 4 on the hunger scale), you won't be physically able to compensate for eating those additional snack calories, and you'll put on weight.

To feel hungry at snack time, you'll need to decrease the size of your meals. If you are used to eating large meals and like the feeling of fullness, this will require an adjustment. Don't worry about being hungry just a few hours later: that's the goal. While the smaller meals may not make you feel as *full*, they may actually be more *filling* than a large one. That's because a large meal causes the roller-coaster effect whereby glucose levels rise sharply and then drop suddenly, causing feelings of hunger just two to three hours after the meal.

Pick Satisfying Snacks

Appendix H is filled with a long list of snack ideas that will satisfy your hunger rather than tempt you to overeat. These are snacks that contain both protein and carbs; many of them are also high in filling fiber. Eating high-carb sweets and salty snacks between meals, for many of us, is just an invitation to overindulge. In one study, people were given 300 calories of their favorite snack foods (chips, ice cream, candy, and fries) to eat every day for two weeks. Afterwards, both normal and obese women reported not liking it as much. Yet while the normal weight women ate less of it, the obese women did not reduce their consumption. So, snack on foods that satisfy you but don't encourage you to overindulge.

Plan for Small Portions

We tend to eat more when larger portions are served. Probably no one has done more research in this field than Dr. Wansink and his team. Over and over again, he has shown that the more people are served, the more they eat, even when they think they are in control. This was true for many types of foods including soup, popcorn, and snack foods. Many of these studies are described in his book *Mindless Eating: Why We Eat More Than We Think We Do*.

In one study, undergraduates were given four 100-calorie packages of crackers or one 400-calorie package of crackers while watching television. The average participant ate 25% less when given four 100-calorie packages. This amounted to less of a difference in normal weight participants and a whopping 54% decrease by those who were overweight.

The good news is that smaller portions can make you feel equally as satisfied as larger portions. Mostly normal-weight young adults were presented with a small mid-afternoon snack totaling 195 calories or a large snack totaling 1370 calories of the same three foods: chocolate chips, apple pie, and potato chips (of course not all of it was eaten). Those served the smaller portions reported similar satisfaction of hunger and craving 15 minutes later as those served the larger portion, even though they consumed an average of 103 calories less. Other people, participating in a computer experiment, were offered unlimited consumption of candy. Interestingly, they ate the same number of *pieces* of candy whether they were full pieces or half-sized pieces (but the half-sized pieces added up to half the calories).

So, if you're going to snack, it's a good idea to buy smaller packages containing smaller items. For example, don't pack a 200-calorie bar if you only want to eat 100 calories. If you can't find snacks in 100-calorie portions, portion and repackage them yourself.

Overweight and obese individuals have a more difficult time incorporating snacks into the day's intake, but by eating less at meals so they are hungry at snack time it's quite possible for them to experience the benefits of adding snacks to a three meal-a-day plan. The key is that snacks must be eaten only in response to hunger and not out of convenience.

EATING PATTERN OPTIONS

While eating three evenly spaced meals improves energy, memory willpower, and health, eating smaller, more frequent meals is helpful to keep your eating under control (to avoid getting overly hungry) or for individuals with higher calorie needs (such as children and active individuals).

Here are some suggested eating patterns that might work for you. Each tip helps to REBOOT your energy by dividing calories more evenly throughout the day in alignment with how you burn them. Keep in mind these calorie splits do not have to be kept firm; always listen to your body and eat when it needs fuel.

• **Three square meals:** This is a good approach for sedentary individuals and those who tend to overindulge when exposed to food, especially in the evening. Instead of banking most of the day's calories in the evening, this approach spreads calories more equally throughout the day (such as 7:00 a.m., 12:00 noon, and 5:00 p.m.). Split your estimated calorie needs more evenly among the three meals. If you're keeping to 1500 calories a day, keep each meal to around 500 calories. No more skipped breakfasts or skimpy breakfast and lunches.

- **Goûter style:** This pattern of eating is helpful for people who eat a late dinner. To prevent getting overly hungry (and overeating), eat like the French and add a planned afternoon snack around 3:00 or 4:00 in the afternoon. Divide your total calories by four, but feel free to modify this slightly to meet your personal preferences and hunger level. For example, if your goal is to eat 1500 calories a day, think about 400 calories for breakfast, 400 calories for lunch, and 400 calories at dinner. Then, enjoy a 300-calorie mid-afternoon snack.

- **Three + three:** For those who enjoy eating three solid meals a day but need just a little snack to control their appetite and prevent overeating at the next meal, try eating three smaller meals plus three planned snacks. To do this, divide your total calorie needs by four. For example, a 1600-calorie-a-day plan would include three meals of 400 calories each and 400 calories for snacks. Then, divide the allotted 400 snack calories among the three daily snacks (about 100-150 calories each). Or, if you have one larger gap, you might opt instead for one 200-calorie snack and two 100-calorie snacks.

- **Six mini meals:** For athletes with higher calorie needs, larger snacks are in order. For this group, it's best to eat six smaller meals evenly spaced throughout the day. Figuring 3000 calories a day, divide total calories by six and enjoy six 500-calorie meals. Sometimes this is as simple as eating half of a restaurant sandwich at lunch and saving the remaining half for a mid-afternoon mini meal.

- **Nibbling:** While there's no energy benefit to eating more than six times a day, some very active individuals, like ultra-endurance athletes burning 4000–5000+ calories a day, like to fuel their activities every couple of hours with nutritious, well-balanced foods. Because of the increased food exposure, eating often also requires regular flossing and brushing to prevent cavities. This nibbling style of eating is not physically or psychologically very satisfying for those with lower calories needs because frequent tiny meals disrupt the ghrelin-insulin relationship, which prevents one from feeling full.

Timing of Meals

Meals should be evenly spaced throughout the day. While there's no reason to avoid eating a small evening snack, large meals can disrupt sleep, so they should be avoided during the three hours before bedtime. This three-hour rule is also a good idea if you have acid reflux.

8

Consider the Fuel Mix (aka What's On Your Plate)

Okay, I've thrown a lot of information your way, and you're still here. That's good! I'm proud of you. But I know some of you just want the answer to the question almost everyone asks me: What is the best diet for losing weight and keeping it off? It's a simple question. Why can't there be a simple answer?

The truth is, just about all those fad diets work to get the weight off – at least temporarily. (If they didn't work, why would they become a fad?) Even if you're not counting calories, when you cut out entire categories of foods, you end up eating fewer calories. And when you eat fewer calories than your body needs, you lose weight. Now, if you want to make sure that the weight loss is from fat (and not muscle) and that you keep it off, *plus* keep your energy up, then you'll need to look at the food on your plate in an entirely different way.

To REBOOT your energy level, you'll need to eat foods that prevent you from feeling hungry or deprived and that contain the nutrients to energize you all day long. I've already discussed how important it is to eat the right amount of fuel and how to space your eating evenly throughout the day. Now it's time to talk about *what* to eat.

Marcia was having a hard time losing weight and complained she was always too tired to exercise. Her diet was based on foods selected for their lower calorie and fat content. She shunned high-fat foods such as meat, nuts, peanut butter, and cheese. When Marcia found out that almond milk had half the calories of skim milk, she made the switch. When she snacked, she chose 100-calorie low-fat snack packs.

Paul complained of lack of energy, too. He was training for a half marathon and found himself crashing during the longer runs. Paul was following a high-protein, low-carbohydrate diet consisting of mostly meat and green vegetables.

In both of these cases, even though the diets seemed balanced, they were not effective in delivering the nutrients needed to maintain energy: protein, carbohydrates, and fat.

THE THREE CALORIE-CONTAINING NUTRIENTS

The Institute of Medicine recommends consuming a wide range of the calorie-containing nutrients to decrease the risk of chronic disease and provide adequate intake of other nutrients, such as vitamins and minerals. The three calorie-containing nutrients (and their recommended proportion of the diet) are:

- **Protein:** 10-35% of calories
- **Carbohydrates:** 45-65% of calories
- **Fat:** 20-35% calories

But you don't want to just survive; you want to thrive. This chapter narrows down those recommendations to a fuel ratio that best provides you with the energy you need to move, concentrate, stay alert, control your moods, and maintain focus on what's important in life. This fuel ratio will also help you have a healthy weight and body composition, too.

As we discuss each of these nutrients, keep in mind that you can't change the amount you eat of only one nutrient without changing the others. When you lower how much you eat of one, you will end up eating more of another. For example, when you increase protein, fat intake generally goes up, while carb intake decreases. This chapter will help you keep a healthy balance by giving you general information on how to plan your meals and snacks. Specific meal and snack ideas can be found in Appendix E-H. If you need a more customized eating plan, contact a registered dietitian nutritionist (RDN) in your area by visiting www.eatright.org and click on the "Find a Dietitian" link.

PROTEIN

Protein, essential for repairing the body and building muscle, is composed of tiny parts called amino acids. Much like the way tinker toys (wooden sticks and spools from our childhood) can be rearranged to form multiple designs, combining different amino acids together form distinctive proteins in our body. Protein is found in both animal sources, such as chicken, beef, eggs, seafood, fish, milk, yogurt, and cheese, as well as plant sources including beans, nuts, soybeans, and tofu. Animal products, as well as soy, contain all ten of the essential amino acids and are referred to as complete proteins. The other ten nonessential amino acids can be provided in the diet or can be created from the ten essential amino acids. Plant sources of protein are often referred to as incomplete proteins because they're missing one or more of the essential amino acids. These are still healthy sources of protein because a varied diet will provide all the essential amino acids within the day.

Benefits of Protein

At last count, I had 3,154, 288 freckles on my body. Ok, that's an estimate; I haven't really counted. But you get the point: I have a lot of freckles, and none of them were there last week. Sure, I had freckles then, but not the same freckles as I have today. This example is a visual of how our DNA programming works. On average, about 1–2% of our body breaks down every day and needs to be rebuilt. This includes not just skin cells, but bone, muscles, liver, heart, hair, nails, and every other cell in the body. Proteins also make up the antibodies that fight infection, enzymes that digest food, red blood cells that carry oxygen, and the insulin that controls blood glucose levels. And, if you've been exercising with the goal of building more muscle, you might need additional protein. Other benefits of eating adequate amounts of protein include:

- **Promotes satiety:** Calorie for calorie, protein is the most satiating of all the nutrients, something that can actually be seen on a functional brain MRI. Interestingly, incomplete plant proteins such as those found in plants are considered more satiating than complete proteins from animal sources. Because protein is filling, including the right amount in a meal may mean eating fewer calories. So, instead of eating a carb-only meal consisting of a salad or pasta, consider adding lean protein.

- **Becomes fuel or fat:** Glucose from carbohydrate is the preferred fuel for the brain and red blood cells. If you don't eat enough carbs, protein is broken down and used to maintain normal blood glucose levels. If you want to ensure that most of the protein you eat goes into maintaining body protein or building muscle, you need to eat enough carbohydrate calories to "spare the protein." On the other hand, if you eat *more* protein than your body needs, the excess amino acids cannot be stored. What isn't needed is turned into fat.

- **Stabilizes plasma glucose:** While carbohydrates are the main determinant of how high blood glucose levels rise during the first two hours after a meal, adding protein to a meal slows this rise by delaying the stomach's ability to empty carbohydrates. (Adding protein to meals has also been shown to improve glucose levels in individuals with type 2 diabetes.) Amino acids from protein also stimulate the secretion of insulin, which increases protein synthesis and decreases the rate at which the body breaks down protein.

- **Increases energy expenditure:** About 10% of the calories we eat are used to turn food into fuel (referred to as the thermic effect of food), but some nutrients are processed more efficiently than others. For example, while only 0–3% of calories are used to process dietary fats, 20–30% of the calories in protein are used for that process. This increase might be due to the fact that the body has no storage capacity for protein and thus it needs to be used immediately to build or replace protein, changed to glucose (gluconeogenesis), or stored as fat.

- **Retains more muscle mass during weight loss and maintenance:** Weight loss never comes from 100% body fat; typically, about 15–20% of total weight loss comes from loss of muscle. Higher-protein diets reduce this loss of metabolism-boosting muscle mass during weight loss and keeps the resting metabolic rate up, which makes it easier to keep the weight off.

- **Improves bone health:** The body's pH (a measurement of acid/base) must be kept within a very narrow range, and dietary protein (especially animal protein) is a source of acid. To buffer this acid load, the body uses calcium. Because 99% of the body's calcium is in the bones, there was once concern that high-protein diets could weaken bones. But this acid load is not a significant factor in those with normal kidney function; in addition, fruits and vegetables can buffer the acid effect. While dietary protein does increase the amount of calcium in urine, it also increases how much is absorbed from our food. Bone is 50% protein, and 8–10% of bone is rebuilt every year, so getting adequate protein (along with adequate calcium) actually *decreases* the risk of osteoporosis. Protein also increases the circulating concentration of insulin-like growth factor, which is important for bone growth. Lastly, because a 10% weight loss can lead to up to a 2% bone-mass-density loss, this higher-protein approach may even help to maintain bone mass during weight loss.

HOW MUCH PROTEIN IS ENOUGH

When you review the upcoming list of protein foods, you'll realize that most of us meet the Recommended Dietary Allowance (RDA) of about 50 g of protein (46 g for women, 56 g for men), enough to replace daily protein losses and stabilize blood glucose. But consuming about twice this amount (80–120 g) may improve energy, satiety, muscle building, and maintenance of muscle mass during weight loss. There's rarely a need to eat more than 150 g per day, and eating higher amounts may even be harmful.

While protein needs are greater for athletes than for sedentary individuals, athletes probably don't need more than they are currently eating. The American College of Sports Medicine's position statement suggests protein intakes for athletes of 0.5–0.8 grams per pound of body weight (on the lower end for endurance athletes and on the higher end for body builders). So, a 160-pound runner would require around 80 g protein (160×0.5), while a 200-pound body builder might need as much as 160 g protein (200×0.8). The reason athletes don't need any more than that is that muscles are actually only 17% protein; most of the remaining weight is water. That means a pound of muscle (454 g) contains just 77 g protein, which is easy enough to get from the protein amounts recommended above. But simply downing high-protein shakes will not build muscle; you have to do the work to stimulate muscle growth.

Maintaining Muscle Strength

Maintaining strong muscles is important because muscles are the powerhouses of the body. The more muscle we have, the more calories we can eat without gaining weight. If you are working out *and* eating adequate protein, but your muscle mass isn't where you think it should be, take a look at what else you eat. Without adequate carbohydrates, the protein you eat will be broken down into glucose to fuel the brain and red blood cells and won't be available for muscle building.

Even if your goal is to lose weight, it's important not to cut calories too low. The body's priorities are always to 1) provide fuel for the brain and 2) replace normal daily protein losses for critical needs such as enzymes, hormones, antibodies, and red blood cells. Only after all these needs are met will the protein go toward building and maintaining muscle mass.

The Best Time to Eat Protein

After eating protein, the increase in blood amino-acid concentrations is complete within 3 hours. The more protein you eat, the higher the amino-acid concentration in the blood, but that doesn't translate into more usable proteins. After 20–30 g protein, muscle protein synthesis becomes saturated. Therefore, it's important to spread protein consumption throughout the day and eat it at every meal, including breakfast. If you eat 25 g protein at each of the three main meals, plus a bit more during snacks, you can easily consume 80–100 g of protein every day. Or, keep your meals to 20 g protein if your snacks tend to be higher in protein. Athletes can meet their increased protein needs simply by eating more than three times a day; consuming 25 g of protein six times a day provides 150 g of protein.

Unfortunately, most of us tend to concentrate our protein consumption to the afternoon and evening hours, eating little or no protein earlier in the day. This translates to daytime meals that aren't filling and evening meals that offer more protein than the body can handle.

Measuring Protein

If you're wondering what 20–30 g protein looks like, remember this: animal meat about the size of a deck of cards weighs about 3 ounces and contains about 21 g protein. One scoop of protein powder (whey, casein, soy, or egg) contains around 20–25 g protein, too. The portion size for other proteins is more variable. Each of the following foods contains about 7 g protein (be sure to read the label on packaged foods for more specific information). To reach 20–30 g protein, aim to eat three servings (examples listed below) at each meal:

- 1 large egg or 2 egg whites
- 1 ounce cheese (1 sandwich slice)
- 1 cup (8 oz) cow or soy milk
- 1 cup yogurt
- ½ cup Greek yogurt
- ¼ cup cottage cheese
- 1 cup bulgur or quinoa
- ½ cup beans (kidney, black, pinto, or red beans, and lentils, chick peas, or split peas)
- 1 serving higher-protein cereals such as Kashi Go Lean cereal
- 1 slice sprouted grain bread
- 1 ounce seitan (wheat gluten)
- ¼ cup soybeans or edamame
- ¼ cup tofu or tempeh
- 2 tablespoons peanut or almond butter
- ¼ cup shelled almonds, peanuts, pistachios, pecans, walnuts, or cashews
- ¼ cup sunflower, pumpkin, flax seeds, chia seeds, or pine nuts
- 1 veggie patty (generally in the range of 7–10 g protein)

While soy protein meets protein needs as effectively as animal sources, the other vegetable proteins may not provide all the ten essential amino acids in one food. While it was once thought that it was necessary to eat complementary vegetable proteins at the same meal (such as beans *with* rice), there's no need to be that strict. Eating an assortment of plant foods throughout the day works to provide all essential amino acids to meet protein needs. Therefore, you could eat beans at one meal and rice at another, if you wish.

When Protein is Too Much

There is no benefit to eating more protein than the recommended amounts mentioned in REBOOT. The excess is simply converted into glucose for immediate fueling needs or stored as fat. Eating a diet that is higher in protein on a regular basis can also manifest itself with symptoms including general weakness, headache, muscle cramps, and GI issues, and may cause some health problems including:

- **Kidney issues:** The process of converting amino acids from protein into glucose for fuel or fat produces by-products including urea, which are eliminated through the kidneys and requires more water to dilute these substances. Although most studies show that healthy individuals suffer no kidney harm with moderate protein levels, the elderly and individuals with obesity, metabolic syndrome, and diabetes are more susceptible to kidney disease and should not consume more than 20% of their calories from protein (or more than what's recommended in REBOOT). Regarding the risk of kidney stones, the Institute of Medicine concluded that there is no clear evidence that high protein intake increases risk.

- **Cardiovascular disease:** The concern for heart disease stems from the fact that an increased protein intake tends to be from animal proteins, which are higher in saturated fat and may lead to a rise in bad LDL cholesterol, cortisol, and CRP (indicating inflammation) levels. This is a good reason to select lean animal and vegetable protein sources such as soy, beans, lentils, and nonfat dairy, or go completely vegetarian.

- **Ketosis:** My major concern about eating too much protein is that it translates into not getting enough glucose from carbohydrates. Diets containing less than 100 g of carbohydrates causes ketosis which can cause nausea and bad breath. Though the body typically burns about 50% fat and 50% glucose, it's flexible. If you don't eat enough carbohydrates, the body adjusts by burning a greater percentage of fat (which includes fat in the diet, not necessarily body fat…unless you're eating fewer calories than you need). After about three days, some of these fatty acids are changed into ketone bodies as a secondary fuel source. Your heart, liver, resting muscles, and fat cells can burn either fat or fatty acids as a fuel. While the brain can't burn fat (fat can't get past the blood-brain barrier), it can slowly adjust to burning some ketones as fuel. The brain does adapt somewhat, but not completely. After three days of fasting, ketones represent about 17% of the brain's glucose needs. After a 40-day fast, one-third of glucose needs are still fed by glucose. Ketones won't fuel the red blood cells; they still require another 200 calories of glucose a day. Eating more carbohydrates allows for an overall healthier diet

• **Nutrient Deficiencies:** Very-high-protein (and low-carbohydrate) diets lack many healthy foods such as fruits, vegetables, and grains, which are rich in vitamins, minerals, and fiber essential for overall health. As you'll see in the next chapter, you'll never reproduce the same good nutrition by taking a multivitamin pill instead of whole foods. Carbohydrates are the only way to create liver and muscle glycogen, which we'll discuss more shortly. Finally, there's no need to cut out carbohydrates because these foods add good-tasting variety to the plate.

CARBOHYDRATES

Carbohydrates include everything from healthy sources such as milk, fruit, beans, and whole grains to the empty calorie variety like cookies, cakes, and soda. While there are many different types of carbs, once they make their trek through the GI tract and travel to the liver, most are broken down into glucose. Skimping on carbs doesn't make sense from an energy perspective because 50% of our body's fuel comes from glucose. Although we can make glucose from protein, that process is inefficient and provides a lot of waste products that have to be eliminated from the body.

Benefits of Carbohydrates

While we can *ineffectively* make glucose from protein, eating adequate carbohydrates offer many benefits including:

• **Improves energy, mood, willpower, focus, and concentration:** Keeping blood glucose levels in the normal range makes us feel better and even reduces the perception of effort during physical or mental work.

- **Critical for brain and red blood cells:** Glucose from carbohydrates provides the fuel for much of the body for the first two hours after our meals. In addition, carbohydrates replenish our liver and muscle glycogen levels. We rely on liver glycogen to fuel our brain and red blood cells between meals. Without glucose or glycogen, the body has no other option than to transform protein from meals (or muscles) into glucose. Fueling the brain and other critical parts of the body is always the body's first priority.

- **Muscle endurance:** Only carbohydrates can replenish glycogen stores. During exercise, the body converts to burning mostly glucose from muscle glycogen. We'll discuss this in greater detail in Chapter 13, but adequate muscle glycogen stores allow the body to workout much harder and longer than when glycogen stores are depleted.

- **Provides great tasting variety for your palate:** There's no reason to skip these valuable sources of vitamins, minerals, and fiber.

Carb Fallacies

Unfortunately, carbs have been demonized and blamed for weight gain when it's actually excess calories of *any* kind that pack on the pounds. Besides, high-calorie foods including cookies, cakes, ice cream, and pies are often thought of as carbs, but in fact, fewer than half their calories come from carbohydrates; most of the calories in these foods come from fat. Like protein, carbohydrates contain just four calories per gram, but fats contain nine. So, it's the fat that makes these foods so fattening, not the carbs. The key to being energized is knowing which types of carbs to eat, when to eat them, and in what amount.

Daily Carb Requirement

You already know your caloric need from Chapter 5. Because 50% of the body's fuel comes from glucose, aim for 50% of your calories to come from carbohydrate, as shown in this chart. Because the Institute of Medicine recommends that 45–65% of calories come from carbohydrate, feel free to customize the recommendation in this chart slightly based on what feels good to you. For example, endurance athletes need more carbohydrate to fuel their muscles. Though, even if you're limiting your calories, don't eat fewer than 150 g carbohydrate per day. This meets the basic needs of the brain and red blood cells.

Calories	Carbohydrates (g)	Carb Servings/day
1200	150	10
1500	190	13
1800	225	15
2000	250	17
2500	310	21
3000	375	25
3500	440	29

Counting Carbs

It's easy to find out the carbohydrate content of the foods you enjoy. If it's a packaged good, read the nutritional label for carbohydrates per serving and compare it to your serving size. While some packages look like single servings, they may contain two to three servings. Many restaurants offer nutrition information online. Apps including MyFitnessPal are also a source for nutrition information. For simplicity, each of the following foods contains about 15 g of carbohydrates:

Fruit

- 2 smaller pieces of fresh fruit (figs, plums, or tangerines)
- 1 small piece of fresh fruit (apple, banana, pear, peach, or orange)
- Half of a large fruit (grapefruit)
- 1 cup fresh fruit (berries, cubed melon)
- 12 cherries
- ½ cup no-sugar-added canned fruit (applesauce, sliced pears)
- 2 tablespoons raisins or ¼ cup other dried fruit
- ½ cup fruit juice

Vegetables

- ½ cup starchy vegetables (corn, peas, potatoes)
- ½ cup spaghetti sauce
- 1 cup winter squash (acorn, butternut)
- 15 French fries
- 1½ cup of most other vegetables (including broccoli, carrots, green beans, tomatoes, and zucchini). There's no need to count smaller amounts of these vegetables, nor the carbs in lettuce, because you'd have to eat more than 10 cups of lettuce to obtain 15 g carbohydrate.

Grains

- 1 ounce bread (1 slice of bread, tortilla, or small roll or ½ pita, English muffin, or hamburger bun, or ¼ large bagel)
- ½ cup beans (kidney, black, split, or blackeye peas)
- 1/3 cup baked beans or rice
- ½ cup oats, grits, pasta, barley, or bulgur
- ½ cup bran cereal, shredded wheat, sugar-frosted cereals
- ¾ cup flaked cereal
- 1 cup puffed cereal
- 6 small crackers
- Breading on a portion of chicken, fish, beef, shellfish
- 2 pancakes (4 inches across)
- 3 cups popcorn
- 2 rice cakes
- 2 taco shells
- 1 ounce chips (about 15 potato chips or 10 tortilla chips)

Dairy

- 1 cup milk
- 1 cup no-sugar-added yogurt
- ½ cup yogurts with added sugar

Other Carbohydrates

- 1 cup soup
- 1 Tablespoon jelly, jam, apple butter, sugar, honey, or pancake syrup
- 2 Tablespoons liquid creamer
- 1 ounce of sweet snacks such as two small cookies (Oreos, Chips-A-Hoy, or Milano) or one medium-sized cookie (Pepperidge Farms Chocolate Chip)
- 2-inch square unfrosted cake or brownie
- ½ doughnut
- 1/12 piece of pie
- ½ cup ice cream or pudding
- ¼ cup frozen yogurt, sherbet, or sorbet
- ½ cup soda
- 1 cup lemonade, sweetened tea, Gatorade, or Powerade
- Candy (½ peppermint patty, 9 gummy bears, 2 caramels, 5 Hershey kisses, or 8 chocolate-covered almonds)

Putting It All Together

With the REBOOT approach, there's no need to prepare different food for everyone in the family. You can plan meals with the appropriate amount of proteins and carbs, in one of two ways. If you're a meat eater, select your protein choice first and then add an appropriate amount of carbs including fruit, potatoes, rice, cooked vegetables, milk, or possibly even a dessert (or use some of those calories for a glass of wine or beer – more in chapter 10). If you don't eat much meat or other protein-rich foods, first figure out what carbohydrate source you're in the mood for, then add the appropriate amount of protein. For example, if you're in the mood for salad, start with a base of lettuce and raw vegetables. Three cups of raw vegetables contain about 30 g carb. Then, decide what protein source to complete your meal. This might include cheese or cottage cheese, beans, grilled chicken or shrimp, or a cup of Greek yogurt.

Each meal should contain 20-30g protein, plus the appropriate amount of carbs. For energy management, I recommend limiting the number of carbs you eat at one sitting to about 30–75g (2–5 carb servings) for meals and 15–45g (1–3 carb servings) for snacks. While this is not a low–carb diet, it's important not to eat too many carbs *at one time*, otherwise you risk experiencing the roller-coaster effect. No meal will fit these guidelines exactly, but here are some suggested nutrition goals for your meals:

- 300 Calories = 20-25g Protein + 2 Carb Choices (30g carbs)
- 400 Calories = 20-25g Protein + 3 Carb Choices (45g carbs)
- 500 Calories = 25-30g Protein + 4 Carb Choices (60g carbs)
- 600 Calories = 25-30g Protein + 5 Carb Choices (75g carbs)

For example, if you need 1800 calories and 225 g carbs (15 carb servings) per day, and you've decided from the previous chapter to keep to 4 meals a day, aim for 60g carbs (4 carb servings) at the 3 meals plus another 45g carbs (3 carb servings) at your afternoon snack.

Because different carbs are absorbed at different rates, it's a good idea to have the carbohydrates from a variety of sources for a more even flow of energy. For example, the 2010 Dietary Guidelines recommend a minimum of 12 servings of carbohydrate foods throughout the day: 3 nonfat milk servings, 2 ½ cups vegetables, 2 fruits and juices, and 6 servings of grains (with half being whole grain) every day. So, to satisfy 4 carb servings, you might choose 2 slices of whole-grain bread, a piece of fruit, and a glass of milk. If you're craving something sweet, skip one of the slices of bread and have a small brownie.

LOSING WEIGHT ON A HIGH-PROTEIN, LOW-CARB DIET

While people on low-carb diets report good results, including weight loss and improvements in blood pressure, insulin, fasting glucose, and triglycerides levels, these results are no different from any other lower-calorie diet. Although the initial weight loss seems greater on a low-carb diet, this difference evens out over time. In other words, the health changes are from the weight loss itself rather than from simply eating fewer carbohydrates. The major health concern with the high-protein approach to weight loss is the typical increase in animal protein. While the good HDL levels improve, the levels of the bad LDL cholesterol don't.

From an energy perspective, a very-low-carb approach simply doesn't provide adequate glucose, which requires your body to burn protein for fuel. In addition, without enough carbs, there's no way to replenish your glycogen stores that enable you to work out harder and faster to build muscle mass. In fact, this loss of glycogen, which is 80% water, is one of the reasons for the initial rapid weight loss often seen when you first start a low-carb diet. The pounds you lose are water, not fat. And that's why you quickly put back on weight when you add carbs back into your meals. Again, this is associated with the normal, healthy storage of glycogen, not fat.

While adding protein to your diet has benefits, eating too much doesn't add additional benefits. I often hear people say they have a lot of energy on the low-carb approach, but this is not coming from the low carbs per se. It comes from the fact that, in following the "diet," they are now regularly eating breakfast, lunch, and dinner. And, while adding protein aids in satiety, adding larger portions doesn't help further. Again, it's not carbs that are the bad guys; it's excess calories of any type that pack on the pounds.

FAST CARBS, SLOW CARBS

For most us, getting enough protein and carbohydrates at each meal (and not too much) makes a huge difference in energy level. If you're still feeling sluggish, tweak your carb intake by focusing on the type of carbohydrates.

Once digested and absorbed, the body can't tell the difference between the glucose molecules of different carbohydrates. Once eaten, glucose from soft drinks appears exactly the same as the nutritious glucose in beans or apples. Each glucose molecule equally satisfies the body's glucose needs. But, the differences between these sources when it comes to maintaining your health and energy are great. Some carbohydrates are simply more nutritious than others. Beans and apples are chock full of added nutrients, while soda is not. While I do believe it's fine to eat some sugar, let's face it: drinking soda or eating sweets in unlimited quantities interferes with your appetite and prevents you from eating foods with the other nutrients you need (without exceeding calorie needs). Another important reason is that some carbs are absorbed quickly, while others are absorbed more slowly.

Glycemic Index

Although all carbohydrates are digested and absorbed into the bloodstream within the first two hours after they're eaten, some are digested and absorbed faster than others. The faster carbs are digested and absorbed, the higher the blood glucose will spike. The term that describes this rise is the glycemic index or GI.

Low-GI carbs are absorbed slowly, so there's a gradual increase in plasma glucose followed by a slow return back to normal over the two-hour period, promoting more even energy. High-GI carbs rise sharply, and, like a roller coaster (see Chapter 6), tend to fall just as quickly (about 30 minutes after eating), leaving you feeling hypoglycemic. Medium-GI carbs are in the middle.

The GI is not an exact science because the index was determined based on the response of 50 g of the carbohydrates tested on only 10 individuals (and most individuals respond to the same food differently from one day to the next, and different people test differently from one another). In addition, GI is also influenced by the type of sugar, starch, or fiber in a particular food. Ripening, processing, and cooking all increase the GI, too.

The American Diabetes Association recommends that for most people with diabetes, the first tool for managing blood glucose is to count carbohydrates and then use the GI to "fine-tune" blood-glucose management. If counting carbohydrates alone isn't enough to control your glucose and energy levels, try eating foods with a lower GI. Since the GI is also dependent upon what else is eaten at the same time, adding protein and fiber to your meals will help to lower the GI. When eating a carb-only snack, be sure to choose one that's low GI.

Determining the GI of Foods

Using glucose as a score of 100, foods are rated high (greater than 70), moderate (56–69), and low (55 or less). Note that "healthy" foods aren't always low glycemic, and "unhealthy" foods aren't necessarily high glycemic. Here's how foods are generally divided:

- **High glycemic:** honey, ripe bananas, cous cous, rice, rice crackers, pretzels, most bread, gluten-free bread, bagels, potatoes, corn, many processed cereals (including whole-wheat mini wheats), soda, jelly beans, cakes, and fluid-replacement beverages (such as Gatorade or PowerAde)

- **Medium glycemic:** berries, mango, grapes, raisins, oranges, pineapple, slightly underripe bananas, fruit juice, oatmeal, carrots, corn, sweet potatoes, pasta, and whole-grain bread

- **Low glycemic:** most other fresh fruits, milk, yogurt, beans, quinoa, winter squash, bulgur, tortillas (corn or flour), barley, nuts and nut butters, hummus, chocolate, chocolate-covered peanuts or almonds, popcorn, and ice cream

Glycemic Load

Just because a food is high glycemic doesn't mean you should avoid eating it completely. In fact, in Chapter 13 you'll discover that eating or drinking a high-glycemic food is a great way to refuel during and after exercise. In addition, eating smaller amounts of high-glycemic foods doesn't raise your plasma glucose any more than larger amounts of lower-glycemic foods. This is where the glycemic load (GL) comes into play. Glycemic load takes into account both the GI *and* the amount consumed.

For example, you might choose pasta (GI = 65) over white potatoes (GI = 100) because of its lower GI. Yet, pasta tends to be served in much larger portions than mashed potatoes. While an average serving of mashed potatoes contain 35 g of carbs, an average bowl of pasta might contain two cups with 84 g of carbs. To calculate the GL of each of these, multiply the respective GI by the grams of carbohydrate in the serving and then divide by 100:

1 cup mashed potatoes: 100 GI × 35 g carbs/100 = 35 GL
2 cups pasta: 65 GI × 84 g carbs/100 = 55GL

Even though the pasta has a lower GI than the potato, we tend to eat more of it, so the glycemic *load* is actually greater. The GL is useful in predicting the acute impact on blood glucose and insulin responses, but for most of us, it may be easier to simply count carbs at each meal instead. While researchers found two times higher glucose and insulin levels over two hours for high versus low GI meals of the same size, the GL was similar for both the small-sized, high-GI and large-sized, low-GI meal. For more information, the international table of glycemic index and glycemic load values of foods from all over the world can be found at: http://ajcn. nutrition.org/content/76/1/5.full.pdf.

The Benefits of Eating Lower GI/GL Foods

Reducing GI/GL is especially important if you're sedentary, overweight, and at an increased risk for type 2 diabetes because it:

- **Lowers fasting glucose and insulin response:** Low-GI/GL eating patterns work by improving glucose response and insulin sensitivity, which reduces the risk of developing type 2 diabetes. Observational studies show that consuming a diet with a high glycemic load increases the risk of developing type 2 diabetes.

- **Increases satiety and reduces hunger:** Thought to be related to the lowered insulin response, this benefit may also cause one to eat less.

- **Helps improve cognitive performance:** A steady stream of glucose, rather than spikes and drops, appears to help attention, memory, and visual perception. Those likely to benefit are the elderly and individuals with diabetes (because diabetes is associated with an increased risk of cognitive decline and development of dementia).

- **Better fat management:** High-GI foods enter the bloodstream quickly and cause a sharp increase in insulin in an effort to bring glucose levels back to normal. Because the body needs only so much fuel at a time, many of these carbs end up as stored fat.

- **Reduces risk of coronary heart disease:** Consuming low-GI/GL meals may reduce the risk of heart disease by raising HDL while lowering triglycerides and reducing C-reactive protein (CRP), an inflammatory marker that is associated with cardiovascular disease. In addition, a low-GI diet has been shown to reduce the slowing of the resting metabolic rate that occurs with low-fat, high-carbohydrate diets.

Tips to Lower GI/GL

You can easily lower the GI/GL by making some of these changes:

- **Choose whole-grain bread:** Instead of white or even multigrain, select a bread with a whole grain listed as the first ingredient such as 100% whole-wheat bread, pumpernickel, and breads made from legume-based flours.

- **Select sourdough bread:** Authentic sourdough bread contains resistant starch that reduces the glycemic response of the carbs.

- **Eat starchy foods cold:** When you cool starchy foods such as pasta, rice, oats, and potatoes, they produce resistant starch that is found naturally in foods such as dried beans.

- **Eat soluble fiber:** This includes nuts, beans, oats, oat bran, apples, oranges, pears, strawberries, blueberries, carrots, cucumbers, celery, and psyllium fiber.

- **Choose unrefined breakfast cereal:** Rolled or steel-cut oats or low-GI processed cereals such as those containing psyllium husks have lower GI.

- **Modify favorite recipes:** Add fruit, oats, bran (including oat, wheat, and rice), and psyllium husks to lower the glycemic response of your cereal or recipe.

- **Keep it simple:** Milling, processing, overcooking, and cooking at high temperatures increases the GI.

- **Choose baby new potatoes:** These have lower GI than russet and other potatoes. Other lower-GI potatoes are showing up in grocery stores, so check the labels.

- **Eat adequate protein:** To slow the absorption of carbohydrates, keep to the recommended carb portion and add 20-30 g protein to the plate.

- **Vary the carbs:** Choose among the lower-GI carbs such as sweet potatoes, parsnips, or all types of winter squash like butternut or acorn.

- **Add fiber to carbs:** For mashed potatoes with a lower GI, try blending in half sweet potatoes, cannellini beans, or cooked cauliflower.

- **Eat more legumes:** Most beans have a GI under 55. If soaking the beans takes too long, use canned beans (choose the lower sodium versions or rinse well before using). Add to stir fries, chili, soups, casseroles, and salads.

- **Choose longer grain rice:** Look for rice, like basmati, that's four to five times longer than its width. These types of rice tend to be more separate and less clumpy or sticky.

- **Undercook pasta:** Pasta and noodles cooked *al dente* have a lower GI.

- **Substitute low-GI grains:** Instead of rice or pasta, try more nutritious low-GI grains such as barley, buckwheat, bulgur, quinoa, whole-kernel rye, or whole-wheat kernels.

- **Don't over ripen fresh fruit:** Over-ripened fruit has a higher GI. For example, it's best to enjoy yellow-only bananas rather than those covered with black spots.

- **Snack healthy:** Reach for nuts, nut butters, hummus, and bean chips instead of cookies, cakes, chips, or pretzels.

- **Limit portion sizes and vary the type of carbs:** Instead of eating four portions of *one* type of carb, enjoy two to three *different types* of carbs in the same meal. Instead of eating a large sandwich, eat just half and add fruit to the carb mix along with a glass of milk.

- **Mix high GI with low:** If you want a soda or dessert that's high GI, eat a lower-GI meal of beans instead of bread or rice.

- **Limit high-GI foods:** There's no need to completely eliminate high-GI carbs, just keep them at no more than half of your total carb intake. Also, don't consume high-GI foods on an empty stomach, except during and after a hard workout. High-GI foods are absorbed quickly and are perfect for instant fuel or to replace glycogen stores (more in Chapter 13).

- **Don't confuse low-GI with healthy:** Some processed foods such as snack/meal bars are labeled low glycemic but aren't necessarily healthy because they contain excessive amounts of processed sugars and unhealthy saturated fats. Read the ingredient list.

- **No need to eat low GI at every meal:** Eating low GI at one meal can decrease the glucose response of the carbohydrates at the next meal. Eating low-GI evening meals can reduce the glucose response to the next morning's breakfast, even in individuals with type 2 diabetes.

FATS

Fats don't influence blood glucose, so small amounts don't directly influence energy level. But because fat (from both food and body fat) provides 50% of the body's fuel and directly contributes to health, it's important to discuss fats when we talk about energy.

Fats are found in so many more foods than you can imagine. Even if you go completely vegan, avoid high-fat foods such as nuts, olives, and avocados, and never add any oil, salad dressing, or other visible fat to your food, your diet will still contain about 10% of the total calories from fat. How so? Even a vegetable like corn still contains some fat (where do you think corn oil comes from?) and, that's okay because eating a diet containing a range of 20–35% of calories from fat helps to maintain healthier blood lipid levels that reduce your risk of heart disease. The participants in the National Weight Control Survey who have successfully lost weight and kept it off consume 20–25% of their calories from fat, while those living in the Mediterranean region and who eat more fatty fish, olives, olive oil, and nuts tend to eat closer to the top range.

I know 20–35% of calories seem like a lot, but fat calories are very concentrated, so they add up quickly. Consider this: if you take a slice of Italian bread (0% fat) containing 80 calories and add a thin slice of healthy oil or spread (100% fat) containing 80 calories, the topped bread now contains 50% of the calories from fat. So, even though only about 10% of the height of this spread looks like fat, 50% of the calories are fat.

Pros

Fat not only adds flavor to foods, it's essential for life:

- **Certain fats can't be made by the body:** Some fats (linoleic and alpha-linoleic acid) are considered essential because your body can't make them. These fats help us to grow normally, maintain healthy skin, and keep the brain and nervous system functioning normally. A deficiency of these fats severely affects brain and nerve development. This is why it's important not to feed babies nonfat milk during the critical first two years of life. After that, kids eat plenty of other foods that provide these essential fats, so nonfat milk is acceptable.

- **Needed for absorbing fat-soluble vitamins:** Fats help the body absorb the fat-soluble vitamins A, D, E, and K. If you're taking a Vitamin D supplement, be sure to take it with a meal that contains some fat. Otherwise, you won't reap its benefits; you might as well just flush it down the toilet.

- **Improves mood:** Adequate fat may help improve mood because low-fat diets have been shown to have adverse effects.

Cons

On the other hand, eating too many fats can be disastrous to our energy, weight, and health:

- **Energy:** High-fat meals make you feel sluggish.

- **Weight gain:** Eating too much fat can easily pack on the pounds for two reasons: fats contain twice as many calories, ounce for ounce, compared to protein and carbs. Also, fats are less filling than the same number of calories of carbs and protein.

- **Displacing protein and carbs in the diet:** Eating too much fat decreases the intake of essential protein and carbs. In addition, a high-fat diet is often high in saturated fats, which are linked to heart disease.

Because there are only three calorie-containing nutrients, when you aggressively cut back on fat, you'll usually end up eating a larger percentage of calories from carbohydrate. If you choose carbohydrate-containing foods with a higher GI, it may increase triglyceride levels and lower HDL levels.

Types of Fat and Their Impact on Health

Fat molecules are made up of many different types of fatty acids. The healthier fats are rich in monounsaturated fatty acids and polyunsaturated fatty acids including omega-3 fatty acids. The less-healthy fats contain more saturated and *trans* fatty acids. Both saturated and *trans* fats raise bad LDL cholesterol and are associated with an increased risk of heart disease. Keep in mind that no fat is 100% saturated or unsaturated. For example, while olive oil contains 15% saturated fatty acids and 10% polyunsaturated, it's referred to as a monounsaturated fat because the majority (75%) of the fatty acids are monounsaturated. The following list offers suggested portion sizes when adding fats:

Monounsaturated Fats

- 1 teaspoon olive, canola, peanut, and safflower oil
- 1/8 avocado
- 8 large olives
- 4 walnut halves, 6 almonds and cashews, and 10 peanuts
- 2 teaspoon natural peanut or almond butter

Polyunsaturated Fats

- 1 tablespoon flax or chia seeds (rich in omega-3 fatty acids)
- 1 tablespoon pumpkin or sunflower seeds (rich in omega-3 fatty acids)
- 1 teaspoon tub margarine or mayonnaise
- 1 teaspoon corn, sunflower, or soybean oil
- 1 tablespoon reduced-fat tub margarine or mayonnaise
- 1 tablespoon regular salad dressing
- 2 tablespoons reduced-calorie salad dressing

Saturated Fats

- 1 teaspoon butter, shortening, lard, palm kernel oil, palm oil, or coconut oil
- 2 teaspoons whipped butter
- 1 slice bacon
- 1 tablespoon whipping cream or cream cheese
- 2 tablespoon light cream, half and half, sour cream, or reduced-fat cream cheese

How Much Fat to Eat

The American Heart Association recommends getting less than 10% of your calories from saturated and *trans* fats. If you eat animal protein such as beef, chicken, and cheese, you're getting plenty of saturated fat in your diet, so you only need to add 1–2 servings of fats per meal (mostly those that are rich in monounsaturated fatty acids because most processed foods contain plenty of polyunsaturated fat).

If you're vegetarian or vegan, you're probably getting more unsaturated fats from the nuts, nut butters, and soybeans consumed for protein. In that case, you can add some saturated fats to your diet and still stay balanced. My suggestion is to consult a registered dietitian nutritionist at www.eatright.org for a customized eating program.

REBOOT TIPS FOR EATING A HEALTHY FAT BALANCE

It's easy to balance the healthy/unhealthy fats when you keep these recommendations in mind:

- Choose lean meats (beef, poultry, fish, seafood) and keep the portions to 20–30 g protein per serving (see protein list earlier in this chapter)

- Trim excess fat from meat and remove skin from poultry

- Eat at least two servings per week of fish rich in omega-3 fatty acids including salmon, albacore tuna, mackerel, herring, halibut, trout, catfish, and striped sea bass

- Add flax and chia seeds, which are also high in omega-3 fatty acids, to salad, yogurt, and shakes

- Drink nonfat and low-fat milk

- Eat low-fat cheese, cottage cheese, and yogurt

- Use canola and peanut oil for baking and stir frying (they have a high smoke point to hold up to the heat) and olive oil for dipping and drizzling

- Choose tub margarines that contain no more than 2 g saturated fat per serving

- Reduce *trans* fat intake by cutting back on processed foods containing partially hydrogenated vegetable oils in their ingredient list. Even when the nutrition label states zero *trans* fats, realize that U.S. labeling laws permit listing quantities as zero when actual amounts are less than half gram (0.5 g) *per serving*, but it all adds up. Pay attention to products such as stick margarine, coffee creamers, cookies, crackers, doughnuts, and biscuits.

- Avoid movie theatre popcorn. Most contain about a teaspoon of saturated coconut oil per cup of unbuttered popcorn. If you can't resist, at least order a smaller size and avoid the buttery topping.

9

Check the Fluid Level and Energy Boosters

After a solid night's sleep and a healthy breakfast, Kathryn's out the door in time to catch the subway that drops her off a brisk six-block walk from her office. She has an apple with almond butter at 10:30 a.m., a chopped salad with grilled chicken for lunch, and carrot sticks dipped in hummus at 2:30 p.m.

She asks me, "I'm fueling my body appropriately, but at 3 p.m. I'm sleepy, unfocused, and just plain feeling lousy. What's up?"

Maybe it's because she's so focused on what she's eating, it doesn't occur to her that she's had almost nothing to drink all day. And she's not the only one. So many people, by mid-afternoon, have had almost no fluids other than a few cups of coffee. No wonder they feel fuzzy headed.

We are made up of mostly water. When we're born, the percentage is 78%, but as adults we are closer to 60% water. Water has no calories, so it does not provide energy, but because the body has such a high water content, even mild to moderate dehydration can cause mental, emotional, and physical complaints like Kathryn's – even when she's doing everything else right.

FLUID

Studies of men and women with moderate dehydration, around 3% of body weight (common after exercising on a hot day), found a noticeable decrease in strength and speed during exercise as well as increased tiredness, decreased alertness, and higher levels of perceived effort and concentration. Another study reported headache and reduced alertness and ability to concentrate.

But even a mild state of dehydration, as low as 1% of body weight, can increase fatigue, negatively affect mood, and make work (both mental and physical) more exhausting. A study of healthy young women found that dehydration greater or equal to 1% didn't affect cognitive performance but degraded mood, increased perception of task difficulty, lowered concentration, and brought on headache symptoms. A similar study with men found more fatigue during exercise and at rest and impaired mood and cognitive performance, including working memory.

Think about that. One percent represents about one and a half pounds for a 150-pound person. Because two cups of fluid weighs a pound, a mild state of dehydration is just three cups of fluid "low." Can you remember a time that you'd forgotten to drink and then downed a large glass of water? That mild state of dehydration might have been enough to affect your energy, concentration and mood, too.

How Much to Drink

The suggestion to drink according to thirst makes sense, except that many of us aren't good at listening to what our body tells us it needs. Yet, it's impossible to prescribe a specific number of cups of water to drink each day because fluid needs vary based on body size, physical activity, heat exposure, sweat rate, and more. For a starting guideline, divide your weight in pounds by two to estimate the number of ounces of water a day. Further divide the ounces by eight to obtain the number of cups. So, a 200-pound man would need around 100 ounces of water or 12 ½ cups. A 144-pound woman might start with 72 ounces of fluid or 9 cups. This matches the Institute of Medicine's recommendation. Chapter 13 offers more guidance for managing fluid during activity.

Hydrated or Dehydrated: How to Tell

A good way to determine if your hydration level is adequate is to look at your urine. While vitamin C supplements and certain medications can darken the color of urine, a hydrated person should have clear or very light pale-yellow urine. If yours is darker than that, chances are you're dehydrated. And if it's the color of apple juice, you're probably very dehydrated. It's easy to get dehydrated, which is why it's a good idea to keep a glass or a bottle of water by your side and sip on it throughout the day. If you don't keep water handy, you're likely to go too many hours without drinking. And, yes, drinking more does mean more trips to the bathroom, but think of them as strategic recovery breaks.

Alcohol is dehydrating, so it's a good idea to alternate a glass of water with each alcoholic beverage you drink. While caffeine also has a reputation of being dehydrating (and is in the short term), the body adjusts over time, which explains why people who drink nothing but *caffeinated* soft drinks, coffee, or tea don't look like prunes. While I'd much prefer you drink more water, caffeinated beverages (such as coffee, tea, and caffeinated sodas) can still count towards your fluid needs.

CAFFEINE: THE FAKE ENERGY

When we are tired, many of us reach for beverages containing caffeine, be it coffee, tea, a caffeinated soda, or perhaps an energy drink. Unfortunately, caffeine alone cannot give you energy. Caffeine is a *drug* that has been shown to increase alertness but not energy, which only comes from food and beverages that also contain calories. While drinking a cup of black coffee may make you *feel* energized, it cannot provide the true energy your brain and the rest of your body use for fuel. That's why I call caffeine "fake energy." So, if you drink coffee and forego eating, you'll have the illusion of energy, but behind the scenes the body is still scrambling to get the real energy you need by breaking down glycogen stores, and muscle protein, to keep blood glucose levels in the normal range.

It takes caffeine about 30–45 minutes to peak in the bloodstream, so don't keep drinking it until you feel totally alert or by that time you will have consumed too much. Besides, a lot of caffeine isn't necessary; a small amount of caffeine (200–300 mg per day) appears to be safe as a quick-fix energizer. As you'll recall from the list of caffeine at the end of Chapter 3, that's about a small mug or two of coffee. Drinking more than 400 mg brings on heart palpitations, nervousness, irritability, and anxiety in some people.

Caffeine can also increase blood pressure; interestingly, this blood-pressure elevation occurs even as your tolerance to caffeine increases. And, remember the average four-hour half-life of caffeine discussed in Chapter 3. Caffeine can prevent you from getting a good night's sleep long after you think the caffeine is gone from your bloodstream.

How to Use Caffeine Therapeutically and Strategically

If you're a big caffeine user, keep in mind that when you regularly drink caffeine all day, you won't dramatically feel its effects. Rather, the contrary: you become tolerant to its effects. If you really want to feel the effects of caffeine, become caffeine-free (or as close as possible) and then use caffeine *only* when you really need a boost, such as a day you didn't get enough sleep. You'll also find that even a small amount of caffeine will get the job done with increased improved alertness, reaction time, and mood elevation.

Rob was a former professional athlete: 30 years old and still very lean (6% body fat). He also assumed he was healthy until he got his lab work back. His blood glucose was in the prediabetic range, and his cholesterol levels were going in the wrong direction. Energy didn't seem to be a major issue until we talked about his day. He described himself as being a clean eater, which he described as avoiding processed and junk foods. Rob also worked out for more than an hour each morning and estimated that he was burning over 1000 calories for the workout alone. All that sounded fine until I asked him about his caffeine intake. It was three times higher than the safe level of 200–300 mg.

Because inadequate sleep can elevate blood glucose levels, I asked him about his sleep. Turns out he was in a vicious cycle. Excess caffeine was keeping him from getting to sleep. Because his sleep was shorter than he needed, he drank caffeine to keep him going during the day. One of the problems with caffeine is that it tends to decrease appetite. So, while his workout alone burned 1000 calories in the morning, he ate little during breakfast and lunch. It took him a while to change, but he started by ordering medium-sized coffees instead of large. Eventually he reported sleeping better and eating more food during the day and less in the evening; his labs started coming down, too.

Coffee or Tea

In a study of 30 healthy volunteers that consumed water or coffee or tea with different caffeine amounts, caffeine significantly sustained performance compared to water. Interestingly, even when tea was prepared at *half* the caffeine of coffee, it provided similar alerting effects as coffee, but because of its lower caffeine content, the tea was less likely to raise blood pressure, disrupt sleep, or cause the jitters.

ENERGY DRINKS

Energy drinks contain ingredients other than caffeine including taurine, guarana, B vitamins, and sugar. While very little research has been done on taurine (an amino acid), it does appear to increase alertness, though double-blind tests indicate that this effect is mostly due to the caffeine. Guarana is a plant that also contains caffeine, but the amount is typically not included when listing caffeine on the label. And, because energy drinks are typically chugged rather than sipped like coffee, the caffeine rush is more immediate.

Energy drinks often contain B vitamins that also offer claims of increasing energy. Look up these B vitamins in a nutrition textbook and, indeed, you'll find that their roles are to produce energy from glucose. But, hold on: that's not the same as *feeling* energized. We are already quite capable of producing energy. If we weren't, we'd be underweight and malnourished. Remember our excess body fat is evidence of *plenty* of stored energy.

B-vitamin deficiencies are rare. Yet, many of these drinks contain many times more than the RDA or even exceed the Tolerable Upper Limits (ULs) as established by the Institute of Medicine. And, taking more B vitamins than you need won't provide you with additional energy. One of the B vitamins, niacin, in high levels can cause an uncomfortable flushing of the skin. If you're worried that you're not get adequate vitamins, I'd much rather you take a high quality complete multivitamin/mineral supplement that has 100% of the daily requirement of a long list of nutrients, rather than a sprinkling of just a few.

Also, remember that energy can only come from calorie-containing foods. So, if the energy drink is sugar-free and calorie-free, there's no way for the body to produce energy from it. If the energy drink contains sugar, then some energy will come from those calories, but a healthier snack would provide longer lasting energy than the sugar found in energy drinks.

Therefore, while energy drinks cause a quick caffeine rush, they don't provide real energy. And, there are downsides to their consumption. The American Academy of Pediatrics states that there's no reason for children and teens to consume these products. Energy-drink-related emergency-room visits have risen over the last few years. While at 10,000 in 2007, visits in 2011 were nearly 21,000. These visits are not just from the energy drinks themselves; many young people are concocting a dangerous combination by mixing energy drinks with alcohol. It's best to drink moderate amounts of caffeine from coffee or tea rather than using energy drinks.

DIETARY SUPPLEMENTS AND OTHER ENERGY-PROMISING AIDS

If you have ever wandered through the supplement aisle looking for a good source of energy, realize you're not going to find it there. Vitamins and minerals contain no calories and, therefore, no energy. Oh sure, taking vitamins and minerals may help you to *release* energy from food, but only if you're deficient in the first place (and most of us aren't). Taking more supplements won't *release* more energy. If you eat a well-balanced diet, especially with high levels of fruits, vegetables, and whole grains, you probably don't need supplements. There's virtually no evidence that taking them enhances energy. But can they influence your overall health?

Do you remember back in the 1990s when supplements of antioxidants like vitamins A, C, E, and the mineral selenium were all the rage? Many well-designed, long-term studies examined the benefits of their use. These included several large studies with tens of thousands of participants, which found no evidence to support the benefits of antioxidant supplements. In fact, beta-carotene and vitamin E seemed to increase mortality, as did higher doses of vitamin A. Even the trusty once-daily multivitamin supplement got the once over, and an extensive review of 26 unique studies of multivitamin supplements with a total of more than 400,000 participants concluded that there was no clear evidence they had any beneficial effect on health including cardiovascular disease or cancer.

Most active people don't need supplements. Recommendations for vitamins and minerals do not differ substantially from dietary guidelines for the average person. The more active you are, the more calories you eat, and the more likely you are to meet those increased vitamin and mineral needs.

In addition, the Dietary Supplements and Health Education Act of 1994 allows supplement manufacturers to make health claims that may or may not be valid. Manufacturers are not required to demonstrate the safety and efficacy of their products, and indeed, there have even been documented problems with contamination or products not having what the label states it is supposed to contain. If you're going to take a supplement, choose one with the USP (U.S. Pharmacopeial Convention) stamp on the label; these are products that have been voluntarily submitted to the USP Dietary Supplement Verification program and have successfully met the program's stringent testing and auditing criteria. I also subscribe to a minimal-cost website, www.ConsumerLab.com, which offers unbiased reviews of supplements and protein powders.

Supplements may only be necessary for individuals with specific medical or nutritional needs. For example, it's difficult for vegans to get adequate vitamin B12, and many menstruating women, vegan or not, require supplemental iron to replace monthly losses. And, while milk is not the only source of calcium, you may elect to take calcium supplements if you can't get enough in your diet. Because requirements are individually based, advising supplements is beyond the scope of this book; please discuss your concerns with a registered dietitian nutritionist.

10

Eat What You Love

I eat chocolate every day, and I make no excuses for this non-perfect behavior. I used to have perfect eating, back in my teens when I was killing myself with an eating disorder. It's not only okay to not be perfect, I recommend it. I want you to feel absolutely no guilt about allowing yourself to eat small amounts of something that has little or no nutritional value if for no other reason than it just plain tastes good. Aiming for perfect eating is unrealistic and totally unnecessary. In fact, a sure way to fail at any new eating plan is to eliminate all of your favorite foods. Oh, it might work for a while, days, weeks, or even months, but then comes the break down and the overindulging.

Just last weekend I went out to dinner with a group of people. One of the guys was stuffing his face with everything, including drinks, appetizers, and desserts in preparation for the big day on Monday: the start of his new diet. While he said he was enjoying himself, he was eating so quickly that he didn't appear to me to be really enjoying any of it. Unfortunately, that wasn't the first time I've seen that kind of behavior. This "Last Supper" mentality, where you eat all the forbidden foods right before you start the diet, is encouraged as you jump from diet to diet. Then, if you break down and eat a cookie, you punish yourself. Finally, you tell yourself you might as well eat the whole bag so it won't be there to haunt you. Please, stop this *diet-du-jour* mentality and get off this cycle forever.

With the REBOOT approach there are no forbidden foods: you can eat what you want. I'll show you how to enjoy all the good-tasting but not-so-nutritious foods and drinks, sugars, unhealthy fats, and alcohol, in moderation.

SIX STRATEGIES TO ENJOY THE FUN FOODS AND KEEP UP YOUR ENERGY

These strategies will give you permission to enjoy your absolute favorite foods without deprivation or guilt, and without compromising your energy, health, or weight:

1. Give yourself permission to indulge

2. Eat your pleasers, skip your teasers

3. Eat pleasers in moderation

4. Enjoy pleasers mindfully

5. Eat pleasers strategically

6. Eliminate your teasers

Give Yourself Permission to Indulge

Any food can fit into a healthy diet as long as it's consumed in moderation with appropriate portion size and combined with physical activity. But how do you indulge without going overboard? On the physical side, when you eat the right foods on a regular basis to prevent blood-glucose swings (see Chapter 5), your cravings are in better control. But some of our need to overindulge comes from our "Last Supper" mentality. So, it helps to stop classifying foods as good or bad. This simplistic approach fosters unhealthy eating behaviors, so when you finally break down and eat one of those foods you've labeled as bad, you tend to berate yourself as a bad person, which prompts overeating.

But if having dessert at home means that the rest of the cake or pie is sitting around your house calling you like the mythical siren, you need another plan. If you have a hard time controlling yourself around these types of foods, enjoy your favorites while dining out, where it's difficult to ask for seconds. Eating your favorite foods away from home also reinforces that pleasurable foods don't have to be enjoyed in secret.

Eat Your Pleasers, Skip Your Teasers

The secret to eating the foods you love and not feeling deprived is to be discriminating. I coined the terms *pleasers* and *teasers* in another of my books, *Dr. Jo's No Big Deal Diet*. Pleasers refer to the foods and drinks that you love. If you had a buffet of every food known, these are the ones you'd definitely choose first. For me, it's chocolate. Teasers are the foods you eat just because they're around. These are the foods you don't know you want until you see them, like an inviting open bag of chips, mint candies at a restaurant, or the dessert that looks way better than it tastes. The clear difference between the pleasers and the teasers is that if you had a choice, you would pick the pleasers.

Once you've given yourself permission to indulge on occasion, you'll need to identify your pleasers. Sit quietly for a moment and ask yourself what you would choose to eat if it were your last meal. Don't say "everything." If you still can't decide, start by ranking general groups of foods. Which do you prefer: fried, sweet, or salty? Crunchy, smooth, or liquid? Once you identify a group, narrow it down in even more detail, all the way down to specific qualities including perhaps the exact type, flavor, and brand. If you like cookies, identify the exact type that tickles your taste buds. Perhaps it's your mom's homemade butter cookies. I *like* ice cream, but I absolutely *love* a rich chocolate-chip ice cream with tiny slivers of chocolate. You may like fried foods, but perhaps you love only very hot French fries from a particular restaurant. If you don't think you are that picky, think again. It's important to narrow your pleasers down to a few real favorites.

If you're having a hard time narrowing your list, sample each of your favorite foods, one at a time, in a quiet place. Look at the food. Smell it. Pick it up and feel it with your fingers. Take a bite. Roll it around in your mouth and truly taste it. Savor it. Is it as good as you expected it to be?

I used to have a hard time controlling myself around cookies. All kinds of cookies. But, after doing this exercise I found that store-bought cookies really didn't taste that good. Most were dry and crumbly. All of them, even the softer cookies, tasted like preservatives. I decided that they just weren't worth the calories. The best part about identifying my pleasers is that I never feel deprived when I pass up store-bought cookies. I deserve better.

Being mindful of calories can help you make decisions. My guess is that when you go shopping for a house, a car, furniture, or clothing you look at the price tag. We do this because knowing the price helps us make a value judgment about the product, to evaluate if it's "worth it." I want you to think of your calorie needs in the same way: as a budget to spend. For me, I'd rather have four dark chocolates than a small piece of chocolate cake with the same calories. That's the difference between a pleaser and a teaser.

Eat Pleasers in Moderation

Once you've identified your pleasers, plan on treating yourself every now and again. While I enjoy chocolate every day, how often you indulge is up to you. It may have to be less often or in smaller quantities than you typically eat them, but not so infrequently that you feel deprived (or that eventually leads to a binge). Restricting access to these foods increases rather than decreases preference.

The American Heart Association states that 1–2 drinks a day may have health benefits, but having 7–14 drinks on one night is an unhealthy binge. The same goes for food; eating too many of our pleasers is a binge, too. Energy-wise, it's better to have a small amount of chocolate every day than to indulge in a full plate of death-by-chocolate dessert every weekend (even if the total calories add up to the same). Eating too much of our pleasers at one time not only negatively affects our energy, it makes it difficult to fit in all the healthful foods and stay within our calorie levels.

Once you understand your calorie needs for the day, it's easy to work in your favorite foods. I recommend that you keep your discretionary calories (saturated fats, sugar, and alcohol) in the range of 10–20% of your total calorie needs. Ten percent is ideal, but because most of us are currently eating an average of one-third of our calories from these foods, 20% is a good initial goal. For example, if you need 1500 calories to maintain your weight, 10–20% is 150–300 calories a day. If you are very active and burn 3000 calories a day, then 10–20% amounts to 300–600 calories of these pleaser foods.

Personally, I need about 2000 calories a day, and I find it easy to keep my pleasers around 200 calories a day. But, on special occasions I feel no guilt about eating 400 calories' worth. And the good news is that this small amount will not negatively affect your energy level.

Enjoy Your Pleasers Mindfully

Once you give yourself permission to enjoy your pleasers, it's important to savor every bite. And I mean *savor*! Pick the perfect time to indulge when you can actually enjoy the experience, not when you're feeling rushed or stressed. Serve them with a table setting, not paper plates. Turn off the TV and put down the book or magazine. Providing yourself special treatment will not only help you get more satisfaction from the food, you'll actually feel fuller with smaller portions.

Next, focus on the act of eating by taking small bites and savoring the food using all your senses. Because those first couple of bites that are the most pleasurable anyway, you'll actually feel more satisfied (and energized) when you eat these small amounts. After that, there are diminishing returns. Think about it: eating one large serving once a week gives you the intense satisfaction of those first few bites just *once*. REBOOT allows you to enjoy that first bite over and over again by mindfully eating a small amount of treats every day.

Eat Your Pleasers Strategically

Whether your pleasers are saturated fats, sugars, or alcohol, the key to including them in your diet without negatively impacting your energy is to eat them strategically, in small amounts during appropriate times of the day. Here's how:

- **Fats:** Fats are the most calorie-dense nutrient. While fats of any type don't affect blood glucose, it's best to eat small amounts throughout the day, rather than avoiding fat all day then over-eating fat in the evening. Because they don't satiate, eating too many fats at one time is more likely to cause weight gain. So, pick one favorite at a time. For example, if I want French fries, I order the veggie burger (not the burger).

- **Alcohol:** Alcohol is best consumed with a meal to slow down absorption because high levels of blood alcohol can negatively affect your energy level. Because alcohol is a drug, the liver goes to work right away clearing it from your system, ignoring the task of preventing blood glucose levels from dropping. There-fore, it's best to always consume alcohol with foods that contain carbohydrates.

- **Sugar:** Sugars and other high-glycemic foods are best consumed during and after hard exercise or with a meal. Sports drinks, gels, and shots are high glycemic and meant to be consumed during and after exercise because they are absorbed quickly to help maintain blood glucose levels and restore glycogen stores. If your pleasers are high glycemic, enjoy them after a hard workout because high-glycemic foods right after exercise doubles your glycogen stores.

Eliminate Your Teasers

While we recognize that bad habits are the result of doing the same things over and over again, realize that good habits are developed the same way. The longer you give yourself permission to enjoy your pleasers, the easier it gets to avoid your teasers. I remember once when a friend asked me if I liked fried chicken. When I said no, he was shocked. When I thought about that, I realized it's not that I don't like fried chicken, it's just that I decided years ago that it wasn't worth the calories. Given a choice between fried chicken and chocolate, chocolate always wins. And, I deserve the very best.

Once you give yourself permission to eat your pleasers, it's time to come up with a plan to eliminate all those teasers that you currently eat. This plan might include simple strategies like:

- not buying them (willpower begins at the grocery store)

- having an honest discussion with others about having these teasers available

- bringing your own snacks to teaser-fraught environments (like parties, airports, conferences, and waiting rooms) so teasers aren't so tempting

- and (most importantly) making sure you eat on a regular basis so low blood glucose doesn't tempt you to give in like the call of the siren

ADDED SUGARS

Current nutrition labeling laws don't differentiate between natural and added sugars. That's why nutrition labels on the milk container list nearly all the carbohydrates as sugar. But there's no added sugar in plain milk, just natural sugar. Same with fresh fruit. Although the body can't tell the difference between a fruit glucose molecule and a soda glucose molecule (and they both have the same number of calories), fruit has additional nutrients such as vitamins, minerals, and fiber, while soda has none.

Eating a small amount of added sugar will not negatively affect your energy levels. While we are well aware of the sugar we add to coffee and cereal, that's just a small amount of the sugar we eat. The problem comes when too many added sugars, including high-fructose corn syrup, white sugar, brown sugar, corn syrup, corn-syrup solids, raw sugar, malt syrup, maple syrup, pancake syrup, fructose sweetener, liquid fructose, honey, molasses, anhydrous dextrose, and crystal dextrose are hidden in processed foods. In addition to affecting energy level, a high intake of added sugars is associated with more calories and a lower quality diet, which increases the risk for obesity, prediabetes, type 2 diabetes, and cardiovascular disease.

Sugar Facts

But before you start labeling sugar as bad, consider these facts:

- **Preference for sweetness is innate:** Infants show a preference for sweet flavors even at birth. While it's easy to label sugars as addictive, we don't overeat those sweet foods until years later. Food intake is driven by a process designed to make sure we get enough calories to meet our needs. Our satiety signals are not just internal, some are environmental, and many are learned. When we wake up to a morning beverage of soda or always have cookies and candies in the house, it's easy to feel that sugar has control over you. Go back to filling yourself first with adequate and healthy calories throughout the day, and those sweets will stop calling you like a siren.

- **We reinforce this preference:** It's interesting that as we mature, we stop feeding our body when it needs fuel and instead fuel at societally approved times of the day. On top of that, many of us were taught as kids to finish everything on our plate, and we still do as adults. When we reward children with sweets or tell them they can't have dessert until they eat their vegetables, we are teaching them that sweet foods are "better" than the rest of the healthy foods on their plate.

- **Sugar is sugar:** Sugar (sucrose) is made up of one molecule glucose bound to one molecule fructose (50/50 blend). While high-fructose corn syrup (HFCS) sounds like it would be much higher in fructose, it's not. High-fructose corn syrup starts off as corn syrup (100% glucose) and is processed to increase the fructose content to either 42% or 55% (soft drinks are 55% fructose). Though the glucose and fructose in HFCS is free (not bound together like they are with sugar), the absorption rates are similar, as are plasma glucose and insulin responses. That may be because their GI is about the same. Using glucose as a GI of 100, sucrose is roughly 68, and cola made with HFCS is 63. Honey is very similar to sugar with 49% fructose, and agave contains about 90% fructose. One of the concerns with fructose is that it has been shown to raise serum triglyceride, but most research cannot differentiate between the effects of high fructose intake per se and total carbohydrate overfeeding. Therefore, it's best to limit both sugar and high-fructose corn syrup to moderate levels.

- **Liquid sugar isn't filling:** Much added sugar intake is from liquid calories such as sodas and energy/sports drinks. Because liquid calories don't fill us up in the same way that food does, these calories are often in *addition* to the calories we need or eat as food.

- **Sugar may play a role in making us sleepy:** When sugar is consumed with the goal of boosting energy levels, it does so temporarily but then leads to a crash (especially when we're sleep-deprived). If optimal energy is the goal, eat moderate amounts of sugary foods *with meals* or pair a sugary snack with protein.

- **It's easy to overcompensate with no-calorie sweeteners:** While every FDA-approved sweetener is safe to eat or drink in moderation and can help you to lose weight (when used to cut calories), there are several problems with using them. The most common problem is the tendency to overcompensate. In research studies where calories were unknowingly reduced with no-calorie sweeteners, people lost weight. But once they were aware of the change, they ate more of other foods with calories. In addition, when artificially and highly sweetened beverages are drunk all day long instead of plain water, biting into natural sweets like fresh fruit tastes bitter or tart and encourages the desire for something sweeter. Personally, I drink one or two artificially sweetened drinks a day including diet soda and iced tea sweetened with less than a packet per glass. I also don't believe that one type of sweetener is better for you than any other. They are all processed and should be consumed in moderation.

ADDED LESS-HEALTHY FATS

The American Heart Association recommends limiting saturated and trans fats including animal fats, coconut oil, palm kernel oil, and palm oil because they can raise LDL cholesterol, which is associated with an increased risk of heart disease. Healthy individuals should aim for no more than 12 g a day when eating 1500 calories a day, 16 g for 2000 calories, and 19 g for 2500 calories.

The following saturated and *trans* fats should be counted as part of your 10–20% of calories limit for added fats, sugars, and alcohol:

- Stick margarine
- Coconut oil, including movie theatre popcorn
- Processed cookies, crackers, and baked goods including doughnuts
- Fatty meats, including prime rib, sausage, and ground beef
- Fried foods, including French fries, fried chicken or fish
- Full-fat dairy products, including milk, cheese, and yogurt

ALCOHOL

Alcohol is not a nutrient; it's a drug, but when consumed in moderation, alcohol can have beneficial effects. Compared to individuals who do not drink alcohol, moderate consumption (one drink per day for women and two per day for men) is associated with a lower incidence of diabetes and heart disease. One drink refers to a 12-oz beer, a 5-oz glass of wine, or a 1.5-oz shot of liquor. On the other hand, it is not recommended that anyone begin drinking or drink more frequently on the basis of these potential health benefits because moderate alcohol intake is also associated with increased risk of violence, drowning, and injuries from falls and motor vehicle accidents.

And I might add, the recommendation of 1–2 drinks per day does not mean you can save up your daily intake and have all 7 drinks at one time. This would be binge drinking, which is associated with a wide range of other health and social problems including sexually transmitted diseases, unintended pregnancy, and violent crime. Excessive drinking can impair short- and long-term cognitive function and increase the risk of cirrhosis of the liver, hypertension, stroke, type 2 diabetes, and cancer of the upper gastrointestinal tract and colon. Remember alcohol is a drug, and it can become addictive.

Alcohol can also make you fatter because it stimulates the appetite and the body doesn't seem to compensate for the calories. Drinking alcohol before a meal can also lower your resolve to eat healthy or in moderation. Some studies show 20–30% more calories were eaten at a meal when alcohol was consumed before the meal. Because alcohol is a drug and the body can't store it, the liver immediately goes to work clearing it from the body, burning as much as it can as a fuel and turning the rest into fat.

Alcohol affects energy, too. While the liver is busy clearing it from the bloodstream, it can't effectively maintain blood glucose levels, which is especially dangerous if you have diabetes. Remember the brain and red blood cells needs glucose on a regular basis. Between meals, it relies on glycogen and some protein to maintain glucose levels, but alcohol impairs this ability to turn protein into glucose, potentially leading to hypoglycemia. That's why it's important to always eat carbohydrates while consuming alcohol. Do not ever decrease your carbohydrate intake to compensate for the calorie intake from alcohol.

I often go to running races where alcohol is served afterwards. This can be a dangerous combination because both blood glucose and glycogen stores are at their lowest after exercise. Consuming alcohol in this state without carbohydrates leads to hypoglycemia. Of course, the effects are exacerbated because of the dehydration that also occurs from exercise. It's best to rehydrate first with a sports drink and then consume the alcohol with food containing carbohydrates.

DEL

Delete Negative Stress

Cal thrives on the tough cases he takes on as a public defender in juvenile court. The challenges, heartbreak, and legal maneuvering he does on a daily basis make "stress" an understatement, but Cal is energized by this work he believes in. He can sit through hours of dry testimony without missing a beat and takes on the most contentious objections without flinching.

So why, his girlfriend wonders, is he sitting across the dinner table from her parents right now, looking like he's about to fade out?

The thing is, there's stress…and there's *stress*.

The word stress often conjures negative connotations, but stress can also be a good thing. In fact, good stress, such as the birth of a child, vacations, or work on fascinating projects (it's different for different people), can help balance out the ill effects of the negative stress we experience—such as traffic jams, tax audits, or meeting the girlfriend's ex-Marine sergeant dad. While some days may be so crazy that you wish for a day without anything to do, realize that life without any stress would be boring and dull.

Negative stress isn't just something you feel in your gut, it leads to a whole host of physical and emotional ailments, excess weight, and an early death. It can also zap your energy on a day-to-day basis. The REBOOT program helps you understand how to interrupt a negative stress cycle and change your thought process to result in a more healthy response.

11

Break the Stress Cycle

Who experiences more stress: a stay-at-home parent or a high-powered executive? The answer isn't quite as simple as you might think because stress is not determined by the number of hours one works nor the complexity of the work. The stress level we experience is related to the *attitude* we have about our work. Let's face it, if you don't like the work you do, no matter how easy it is, the more stress you're likely to experience.

THE STRESS CYCLE

Hans Selye, the physician who coined the term *stress* described it as the nonspecific response of the body to any demand, whether psychological or physical. Stress can be a real event (like the near-car-accident described in Chapter 1) or something imagined such as when we worry. The body immediately responds to stress with two different and complex body systems that create a sequence of events that can literally save your life, or, if allowed to become chronic, leave you fatigued and ill.

Acute Stress

In that near car accident situation it takes just a split second for the body to release stress hormones including adrenaline and cortisol, which promptly initiate the chain reaction of increased blood pressure, heart rate, and breathing to get sufficient oxygenated blood to the muscles needing to respond quickly to danger. At the same time, the body also releases glucose into the bloodstream to provide the extra fuel that's needed to quickly slam on the brake or swerve out of the way. No matter how fatigued you were before that type of event, your attention quickly becomes sharpened and focused. These normal physiological changes are referred to as the fight-or-flight response because it allows the body to respond faster and with more strength than usual to fight or flee danger, either real or imagined. This is all good.

Chronic Stress

But do you remember how you felt after that near car accident? Most likely, you felt lightheaded, weak, nervous, and fatigued. While the reaction to stress is healthy and lifesaving, if we keep putting ourselves through it over and over again, many times a day, we end up totally wasted.

Of course, not all stress comes from near car accidents. (Well, I hope not!) Sometimes stress is the result of a reaction to actual daily events like the jolt from the Big Ben blare of your alarm clock, dealing with bad traffic, or weather events. Most of the time though, a stress reaction occurs because of psychological reasons including negative thoughts that you just can't seem to stop thinking about. These thoughts could be anything from a running tally of all the things you need to do, worries about your job or health, to simply repetitive annoying thoughts such as thinking about someone who "doesn't understand" or is "driving you crazy." All these thoughts are capable of causing the stress reaction to be played out over and over again. This stress wears you out, and if it goes on long enough, it can leave you feeling like you're at the end of your rope.

Adverse Effects of Chronic Stress

While acute stress causes immediate alertness, when it's over and things calm down, maybe during the drive home after work (or soon after), you'll likely find yourself exhausted and fighting heavy eyelids. This is especially true if you've been attempting to fuel yourself all day with caffeine and sugar rather than getting true energy from eating healthful foods. The physiological and psychological changes associated with repetitive debilitating stress reactions lead to:

- **Physical issues:** Physical issues can include gastrointestinal problems, backaches, and headaches. Chronic stress also increases the risk for high blood pressure, chronically elevated glucose, a weakened immune system, heart disease, and fatigue.

- **Emotional issues:** Emotional issues can include mood swings and irritability or the inability to relax leading to insomnia.

- **Mental issues:** Mental issues can include impaired memory and concentration or impulsivity that can lead to making more errors and more misunderstandings.

Stress is also a significant risk factor for heart disease, the leading cause of death in the U.S. for both men and women. In the InterHeart Study, a case-control study of heart attacks in 52 countries, researchers found that stress and depression were responsible for nearly one-third of the attributable risk, only slightly less than the risk related to a lifetime of smoking and greater than that for hypertension or obesity.

Stress and Weight Gain

Mari asked me how to get rid of her recently acquired belly fat. While she was aware of how genes affect our body shapes, no one else in her family developed fat around the middle at such an early age. Turns out unmanaged stress may very well be playing a role. One of the roles of the stress hormone cortisol is to increase the breakdown of body's stores to supply the extra fuel needed for the muscles to respond in emergency situations. These fuels include stored glucose and fat. But, because most stress is the result of false alarms (meaning there's no real dragon to slay or lion from which to run), the body really doesn't need this extra fuel that is now floating in our bloodstream. It has to go somewhere, so it is turned into fat.

There are two types of body fat: subcutaneous fat (the stuff just underneath the skin) and visceral fat (the dangerous belly fat). Because visceral fat has up to four times more cortisol receptors than subcutaneous fat, unfortunately, more of these stress-mobilized stores turn into visceral fat. That's why people who secrete high levels of cortisol (salivary tests are available) have higher levels of visceral fat, indicated by a waist circumference of more than 35 inches for women and 40 inches for men. In laboratory settings, women with high levels of belly fat rated challenging situations as more threatening more often, performed poorly when trying to execute them, exerted increasingly less effort on them over time, and ultimately, reported more chronic stress in their lives. These women also tended to secrete more cortisol in response to stressful situations than women with less belly fat.

Our physical response to stress may explain why we either eat or lose our appetite after a stressful event. In one study, women who secreted high levels of cortisol ate more on the stress day compared to women who secreted lower levels of cortisol. Those with the higher levels also ate significantly more sweet foods, regardless of the stress level. Another reason people eat more in response to a stressful situation is that as blood glucose increases to help muscles respond, it leaves critical cells starving for glucose, leading to an increase in appetite.

MANAGING STRESS

Experiencing a certain amount of stress is normal in daily life, and failure to respond to stress is pathological. But, it's important to reserve most fight-or-flight reactions for true emergencies, as chronic stress has negative repercussions. Just as computers can only handle so much power at once, the body can only take so much stress before it short circuits. Practice the following guidelines as your surge protector from stressful situations.

Practice (or Project) Positivity

Anytime you gather a few people together, you realize there is no *one* reality. Life is how each of us sees the world through *our* lens of experience, background, and perspective. I realize it sounds so simplistic, but think of how you see the world. Are you a glass half full or a glass half empty kind of person? Having a positive perspective makes all the difference in the world in mood, physical health, and level of success in life. Here's how:

- **Smile:** Putting a smile on your face can change your mood as well as the attitude of the people around you, and it may also keep you alive longer. Researchers rated the smiles of 230 baseball players who played before 1950 (based on pictures in the Baseball Register) and then looked to see how long the players lived on average. Those without smiles lived to an average age of 73, those with a partial smile lived to 75, while those with a full smile made it to 80. So, smile even when you don't feel like it. It just might change your life.

- **Think happy thoughts:** When we're happy, we feel energized, but when we're sad, we drag. Happy brains produce more of a neurotransmitter called dopamine, which makes us feel alert, focused, and full of energy. The good news is that the external world is only responsible for influencing a small amount of happiness; most of it comes from our internal attitude. While success can't buy happiness, happiness can bring success. Happy people get further in life and make more money. So, hang around with happy people, watch happy television shows and movies, and don't watch the news right before going to bed.

- **Laugh:** The muscular exertion required to laugh releases endorphins, those feel-good brain chemicals that boost energy and mood and reduce pain. Laughter is also capable of lowering blood pressure and improving immune responses. When your perspective of the world is in a funk, look to the things that make you laugh, like going to an amusement park, reading something funny, visiting friends, or even watching silly YouTube videos.

- **Spend time with kids:** Children naturally have a more positive attitude. They think almost everything is possible. So spend some time with your kids, nieces or nephews, or just go to the park and watch kids play. When my daughter was young, and I was in a funk, we'd go to this huge play center where both kids and adults were allowed to crawl through tubes and exit on slides that landed you in a tub of colored, plastic balls. It did wonders for my mood and energy!

- **Express gratitude:** Expressing gratitude has been shown to increase feelings of well-being. So, take the focus off you and your worries and thank or compliment someone or simply journal about the things you are thankful for.

- **Volunteer:** When you help other people, it benefits your physical and emotional health, diminishes physical pain, and improves mental health. So, volunteer for an organization you feel strongly about or simply help out a neighbor in need.

- **Adopt an "Oh well, that's life" attitude:** When bad things happen, remember that getting upset is exhausting and accomplishes nothing. In fact, it shuts down the ability to brainstorm for a resolution to the situation. Before reacting or responding, take it down a notch. I try to calm myself by reciting (out loud or to myself) "Oh well, that's life," or "It is what it is." One of my keynote participants nicknamed that last comment as, *iiwii* (pronounced ee-whee). It spread around her office like wildfire causing people to shout "iiwii!" and giggle when small unfortunate things happened.

- **Avoid all-or-nothing thinking:** Nothing is true 100% of the time, except for gravity, taxes, and death. Nonetheless, we continue to use all-or-nothing words to describe many aspects of life. We categorize people and things that happen to us, immediately labeling events as good or bad. Instead, try to remain open to potentially positive outcomes of even the most seemingly negative events. There's always some bad in the good and some good in the bad (even cancer). Joni Rodgers writes in her book, *Bald in the Land of Big Hair*: "In the great barnyard of life, cancer is a manure pile. It stinks, but it makes great fertilizer." It also helps to keep caffeine intake down because excess caffeine increases anxiety, which affects how you'll respond.

- **Look for evidence of the opposite:** It's easy to get caught up in negative emotions after a misfortune. Martin Seligman, the father of the Positive Psychology movement states that individuals with a pessimistic attitude tend to believe bad events will last a long time and undermine everything they do; optimists look at misfortune as a temporary setback and just try harder. When something bad happens, search for evidence that this is only temporary and check out how others have overcome the same or similar setbacks. I've seen people look at a job loss as the motivation to go back to school and ultimately get the job they really wanted, as well as others who have recognized their diagnosis of a disease as the kick they needed to change their lifestyle.

- **Know thyself:** We are all different, and we need different ways to manage stress. For example, extroverts find that being around people gives them energy, while introverts need time alone to reboot. Pay attention to your body's stress signals (such as a shortened temper, out of control eating, or insomnia) as well as what people, things, or situations stress you out.

Control Self-Talk

Henry Ford said, "Whether you think you can or you can't, you're probably right." If we don't think we can accomplish something, we usually don't even try, so nothing changes. If your thoughts are literally strong enough to determine your destiny, it stands to reason that these same thoughts are also powerful enough to affect your energy level. Our thoughts determine much of how we respond to any given situation. To decrease stress levels, take a look at the way you perceive various situations such as these:

- What did you say to yourself the last time you stepped on the scale?
- Do you yell at other drivers even though your windows are up and they can't hear you?
- Do you make comments, out loud, while watching the news on TV?
- If you trip on something, do you call yourself a klutz?
- When you put your foot in your mouth, do you call yourself stupid?
- When someone says something not so nice to you once, do you repeat it over and over to other people and think about it constantly?

How have any or all of these behaviors been working for you? Chances are, not so well. Did that number on the scale determine the rest of your day, or was it your reaction to those numbers? When you yell at other drivers, in your head or out loud, do they change their behavior? Heck, I still can't get my husband to change any of his behaviors, and he loves me; those strangers don't love you. When you take 10,000 steps in a day, does one little misstep really make you a klutz? Even if you tripped 10 times in a day, that is still 1% of the time, which means that 99% of the time you're walking just fine. When someone says something not so nice to you, sure, simple courtesy suggests they keep their big mouth shut, but you heard it only once. What's worse is the 1,000 times you repeated it to yourself and others. Like any habit, the more you repeat it, the more ingrained it becomes in your life. The more you repeat stressful comments, the better chance they have of becoming your reality.

Unlearn Negative Behaviors

Many stress responses are learned behaviors, and this means they can be unlearned. Here are some strategies to help you manage your self-talk so you don't put yourself continually into a stress response.

- **Get the story straight:** Do you remember Emily Litella, one of many characters played by Gilda Radner on Saturday Night Live back in the late 1970s? If you haven't seen them yet, watch some of these hilarious segments on YouTube. In a high-pitched, warbly voice, Emily would recite an outraged rebuttal to an editorial that a TV station had supposedly broadcast. Key to each of these monologues was a simple misunderstanding, often just one word. Once she was informed, she demurely ended with, "never mind." Like Emily, have you ever blown off the handle before getting all the facts?

- **Focus only on what you can control:** When the perceived threat is greater than the perceived ability to cope with the threat, it causes stress. You're likely to deal with this type of situation with thoughts of, "there's nothing I can do." While, it's true that we are often faced with situations we can't control, there's always one thing that we *can* control: our attitude.

- **Don't give free rent to negative thoughts:** Years back, there was a public broadcasting commercial showing a close-up of a women's face berating a child with comments like, "you're no good for nothing, you can't do anything right." It ended with text of how abuse isn't always physical; it's also emotional. Of course, we'd never put up with someone verbally abusing us that way, but how many times do we say the same things to ourselves? That negative language doesn't help others, and it doesn't help us, either. If you're guilty of this, make a commitment to stop. It's important to admit your mistakes but without self-flagellation. Next time you beat yourself up about something you didn't do perfectly, write down what a good friend or relative would say to you, read it back to yourself, and take it to heart.

- **Stop "shoulding" on yourself:** Do you ever scold yourself with statements that begin with, "I *should* have…"? With each scolding of what you should have done or should have said, you beat yourself up unnecessarily. Try using the word *could* instead. The word could offers choices without shame. Sure, there are always a lot of things that could be done, but who says you should? Stick to your priorities. And, as far as dwelling on what others should have done or said, remember you can't control them. They have their priorities, too.

- **Realize that no one can make you mad:** We often say, "s/he's driving me crazy," but in reality, no one has that ability. No one can get inside our head. However, by continuing to repeat garbage thoughts in your head, you'll end up driving yourself crazy!

Stop Worry, Replace with Mantras

As a kid, I was always puzzled when my grandfather said he worried about us. I never understood why. Now, as an adult, I can relate. But really, is worrying productive? It certainly is exhausting.

Realize that it is possible to manage only one thought at a time, so replace a worrying thought with a positive mantra. To do this, change the words you generally use to ones that are still true but positive:

- My friend used to always say, "I hate my job," but in today's bad economy, she's changed to saying, "I have a job, and it pays the bills."

- A neighbor once said, "I used be short, fat, and ugly. Now I'm petite, full-bodied, and don't give a hoot what anyone thinks of my looks."

- A colleague suffered a heart attack in his forties. Now, his new mantra is, "another beautiful day above ground."

Tailor your mantras to be more specific towards your goals. And the more you repeat these positive phrases, the more you will believe them, and positive behaviors will follow.

- Instead of berating yourself for what you just ate, try saying, "I enjoy eating healthy." Yes, eventually, you will start believing yourself, and healthy eating will follow.

- If you're stressed about finances, keep repeating, "I'm saving a little bit every month, and my credit-card debt is coming down." And, it will.

- If you're not good with making cold calls, try saying to yourself, "I follow up with leads on a timely basis." Soon, you'll be living up to this claim.

You know how easy it is for a song to get stuck in your head, so use this same tendency to repeat a catchy melody song as your mantra. When my life gets stressful, I start singing James Brown's "I Feel Good," or I play Pharrell Williams' "Happy." What's your theme song?

Use Your Mind

The brain can't tell the difference between a real event and an imagined one. That's why you jump in response to a scary scene in a movie. Rationally, we know it's not real, but our body still reacts. Dr. Peter Fox at the University of Texas Health Science Center at San Antonio conducted research on the powerful effects of visualization. In several experiments, he attached brain electrodes to athletes to measure their brain activity and found that regardless of whether these athletes were imagining themselves participating in the sport event or really practicing the activity, some of the same parts of their brain were stimulated.

Visualization is widely used among professional and Olympic athletes, who visualize themselves succeeding within their sports, successfully shooting baskets, skating a routine flawlessly, or running faster than ever before. And it works. We can take a page from these athletes and use visualization to deal with stress just as effectively.

Because the body can't tell the difference between reality and fiction in sports or when dealing with stress, we still experience the same response even during imagined situations. These responses include all the negative aspects of stress: high blood pressure, migraines, insomnia, weight gain, and exhaustion. If this is a problem for you, think about getting professional help, and practice these ideas for how to quiet the mind:

- **Take deep breaths:** Try a simple exercise of closing your eyes and taking ten slow, deep breaths to reverse the physical response to stress; it will lower your pulse, breathing, and heart rate.

- **Meditate:** Although meditation is largely rooted in the world's spiritual traditions, practicing it does not require belief in any particular religious or cultural system. Meditation is about becoming mindful of your thoughts and observing them in a nonjudgmental way.

- **Try movement-based meditation:** Qigong, tai chi, and yoga all work to reach a relaxed state through focused breathing, slow movement, and poses. But even something as simple as sitting in a rocking chair can also function as mediation.

- **Use active relaxation:** People who have a difficult time sitting still find repetitive exercises such as stretching, walking, running, dancing, and swimming laps to be relaxing, and perhaps, meditative.

- **Pray:** Quiet the mind through prayer at home or in a house of worship.

- **Use imagery:** There are many CDs and apps that use imagery to lead you to a state of relaxation by helping you find your "happy place."

- **Escape to nature:** Years back, I lived on an overgrown wooded lot. It's amazing how stress relieving it is to chop down trees, but it also relaxing to listen to the sounds of nature. Try soundscape music and get yourself a small water fountain for the office.

- **Practice mindfulness:** Mindfulness is about stopping and being present. Sure, thoughts will continue to pop into your mind. Just think of them as waves rolling in and then dissipating.

- **Journal:** Just open up a blank notebook and give yourself an opportunity to write, non-stop, for a few minutes about your thoughts and emotions to get them off your chest.

- **Get a massage:** The benefits of massage are well documented. A good massage will leave you physically and mentally rejuvenated and relaxed. If you've never experienced one, now is the time to try.

Identify Your Life Purpose

People who live their life's purpose are much happier and more energized. Identifying and living your life's purpose not only increases life satisfaction, but also lowers stress to promote a healthier, longer life. This is because having a purpose motivates us to rethink and reframe stressful situations in order to deal with them more productively. Chicago-based Rush University Medical Center's Alzheimer's Disease Center shows that having a purpose in life helps stave off cognitive decline. To help you define what gives your own life meaning, start here:

- **Don't allow yourself to get bored:** Boredom is enough to make anyone feel tired and lethargic. It might even be deadly. A research study found that people who retire at age 55 were nearly twice as likely to die earlier than those who worked until they were 60 or 65. Even after retirement, it's important to find challenging things to do.

- **Define your life's mission statement:** Having a formal mission statement that identifies your aims and values can help you keep your life on track. My mission statement is to "inspire busy people to stay healthy, sane, and productive while maintaining close, healthy relationships with the people who are important to me." What's yours?

- **Spend time with the people who are important to you:** Deathbed confessions never include remorse over not having worked harder. No job need be so consuming that your important relationships suffer.

- **Discover what energizes you:** This includes evaluating your current job satisfaction, where you live, and the people in your circle.

- **Practice your hobbies:** Too often we forget the hobbies that gave us joy in our earlier years. Hobbies add an important dimension to life because doing them can be energizing and temporarily allows us to forget our worries. So, dust off the piano or put on your basketball shoes!

Improve the Work Environment

Many of us spend most of our time at work. Because work can often be a source of stress and anxiety, it's important to do all you can to make your work environment pleasant for both your mental and physical well-being. There are various ways to control stress at work; some require policy and procedural changes, but there are others you can institute on your own:

- **Set limits:** There are diminishing returns to working long hours. So, honor your recovery breaks, weekends, and vacations. Make sure you go home each evening on time, too; adverse physical and mental health results from working more than 60 hours per week.

- **Add light:** Darkness promotes melatonin production, which makes you sleepy. Bright lights are invigorating, especially in the middle of your workday when your circadian rhythm is at its lowest. If the lighting at your workplace is insufficient, consider bringing in your own.

- **Go back to nature:** Some companies are bringing the workplace to the great outdoors by installing roof decks and patios to help fight winter blues. Having a plant in your office also helps. If you don't have a window, there are many varieties that thrive in florescent office light.

- **Consider ergonomics:** Proper posture reduces the strain on the body. Try a stand-up or walking desk to offer you a break from sitting.

- **Take recovery breaks:** Walk away from your desk every 90 minutes or close your eyes, take a stretch, or go for a walk.

- **Go out for lunch:** Even if you just go to the lunchroom, don't eat at your desk.

- **Have stand-up meetings:** Get rid of the chairs and offer one big standing-height table to help keep meetings short.

- **Leave work at work:** It's not always possible to turn off the smart phones all evening long, but at least make the dinner table sacred time with family, friends, or even for yourself.

- **Have fun at work:** People who have fun on the job are more creative, more productive, better decision makers, and get along better with coworkers. They also have fewer absent, late, and sick days than people who aren't having fun. Look no further than *Fast Company* magazine for ways to have more fun at work. Try hosting a sporting event, organizing a movie night, or adding fun games to the break room.

- **Quiet the noise:** Even low-intensity background noise has been shown to have a disruptive effect on people's ability to learn and process information. White-noise machines can help to tune out office chatter and more.

- **Listen to appropriate music:** Music at the right tempo and volume can boost motivation and make work (and exercise) seem easier.

- **Stop multitasking:** All of us are being overloaded with email, phone calls, social media and more. While doing two things at once seems like a timesaving tool, it's actually less productive because it increases errors. This should be pretty obvious to you if you've ever been called on during on a conference call while trying to read and answer email. The human brain can't successfully perform two actions concurrently. In addition, higher levels of stress hormones are released when multitasking.

REBOOT Your Willpower

We often blame lack of willpower for why we can't stick to our diet, stay on an exercise program, or make the other healthy changes we feel are necessary. These strategies will help:

- **Refresh your willpower:** Willpower is like a muscle in that exercising it too much tires it out. To stave off willpower fatigue, get enough sleep, take strategic recovery breaks, eat when hungry, enjoy your pleasers on a regular basis, and spend time with people, and do things that are fun and important to you.

- **Be selective:** Willpower uses energy in the form of glucose, so be choosy how you spend it. If you hold back speaking up at work, resist the vending machine in the afternoon, and work long hours without taking a recovery break, you're likely to be out of willpower by dinner and pay for it with an uncontrollable urge to dig into second helpings. Instead of using your energy to combat all the little stressors in your life, save it for the things that matter most to you.

- **Believe in yourself:** Willpower is not as finite as we think. In fact, our reduced willpower may be more a result of our *belief* about how much willpower we have, rather than running low on it. When you think you have lots of willpower, you'll be surprised to find out that you actually do.

- **Don't strive for perfection:** Trying to be perfect is stressful – and impossible. No one is perfect! Instead, spend your energy and willpower on the important things that you want to accomplish – and let the other things go.

Develop Healthier Habits

Instead of trying to cut out bad habits, consider that it's easier to replace them with healthier ones. Consider these:

- **Develop new habits one at a time:** Trying to change all our unhealthy habits at the same time never works, especially over the long haul because we fall into many habits automatically, without consciously thinking about them. The more we repeat any habit, healthy or unhealthy, the harder it is to break the pattern. When you decide to change a habit, pick just one change at a time, then give it time to become your new, healthier habit.

- **Give it time:** While we often hear that it takes 21 days for a new habit to develop, that's a fallacy. Some new habits take less than 21 days to develop, but most take way longer.

- **Replace, don't suppress:** Instead of suppressing an unhealthy habit, try to change it to a healthier one. For example, note your cravings and urges and come up with a healthful substitution. If you usually drink soda, switch to diet soda or get up and take a walk instead. Soon the new substitution will become the new habit.

Remember, stress isn't caused by what *happens* to you; it's caused by how you *react* to what happens to you. You have control over your reaction and can choose how you respond. When you practice the stress-management strategies outlined in this chapter, you'll develop the skills necessary to save major fight-or-flight reactions for true emergencies. If you don't control stress, it will control you.

RESTART

Use Movement to Restart the Engine

When my daughter came home from her first day of first-grade, I asked her what class she liked best. She quickly responded, "Recess!" That probably doesn't surprise you. As children, we all loved to move and play, yet most of us have gotten away from it – a huge factor related to our diminishing energy.

Lack of time is the #1 excuse I hear from my audience members. In chapter 12 we discuss how the benefits of movement far outweigh the time; dedicating just a small part of your day in movement can actually increase your energy, focus, and productivity. After covering the benefits of movement, I'll provide six simple steps for moving more – including a list of more than 100 fun ways to move more (most don't involve going to the gym).

If you already exercise you'll want to dive into chapter 13 – how to fuel your movement to make sure you get all the benefits of your workouts. At the end of every yoga practice we do our final pose – savasana or corpse pose. That's where we lie flat on our back and relax. The yoga teacher always prefaces it with, "Now for the most important pose of the class." Early on in my practice I used to think, "How can this be important if it's so easy to do?" But, that's so true for all types of movement – it's not just the time you spend on exercise, but what you do *after*. If you don't fuel yourself appropriately, you may have wasted your time. Chapter 13 shows how simple it can be to rebuild your body stronger after workouts to allow your body to have more energy.

12

Movement for Fun, Fitness, and Energy

If you have gotten away from movement, ask yourself why. Part of the reason may come from answering this simple question: When you were a kid, did you like recess or gym class better? My daughter told me recess was her favorite because recess was on *her* terms and gym class was on *theirs*. Recess was something she *wanted* to do, while gym was something she was *supposed* to do. She said, "At recess you get to play with anyone you want to and you don't have to change your clothes or follow anyone else's rules! I hate other people telling me what I *should* do."

If you have difficulty getting motivated to exercise, perhaps it's because you think of it like gym class with a uniform and a set of rules made up by other people. If you don't exercise because you don't have time, consider that the average person spends about 34 hours a week watching television (and that's not including the programming we view on the computer). Or maybe you think of exercise as hard work. I'm guessing if you perceived movement as fun (like recess), you'd make it a priority. That's why I often refer to exercise as movement; frankly, I think it sounds a lot less daunting than exercise. Whatever you wish to call it, it's important that you just do it.

If you want more physical, emotional, and mental energy, it's critical that you get up and move on a regular basis. This movement includes aerobic exercise that increases your heart rate to build endurance, resistance training that uses weights or your own body weight to increase muscle strength, and stretching to increase flexibility and prevent injury. This chapter covers the benefits of movement and how to fit it into your busy day, along with more than 100 ideas of how to make it as much fun as it was when you were a kid. Of course, you'll need to check with your doctor before starting any exercise.

WHY WE NEED TO MOVE

There are so many benefits of moving more including:

- Improved energy and mood
- Improved fitness for both body and brain
- Enhanced insulin sensitivity
- Longer, healthier life
- Stronger bones
- Burning more fat
- Weight maintenance
- Minimizing muscle loss
- Improved appetite control
- Better sleep quality

Improved Energy and Mood

I have a bumper sticker that reads, "Run…it's cheaper than therapy." It may sound like I'm being facetious, but regular movement substantially improves energy, focus, and mood. In fact, some studies demonstrate that exercise is just as effective as cognitive behavior therapy and anti-depressant medications in alleviating symptoms of *mild* depression. Pairing aerobic with resistance exercise using weights appears to work even better to increase energy and improve mood than aerobic exercise alone. And, high-intensity movements (such as jumping rope or running) appear more effective than walking or other low-intensity exercise.

Adding short bursts of strategic movement can make a major difference in your overall energy and have a positive effect on your job performance, too. Recently, Wellness and Prevention Inc. conducted a 90-day workplace study called Organizations in Motion, which measured the impact of taking short but frequent physical-activity breaks throughout the workday. Those reporting high energy levels increased by 11%, and nearly half of the participants reported increased engagement and focus at work.

Fit Body, Fit Brain

Fitness, at any age, is good for the brain. Kids who are physically fit have improved concentration, learning, and memory, and exercise can slow down the changes that come with age including brain shrinkage and dysfunction. Movement helps the different parts of the brain communicate with each other and to retain what is referred to as "plasticity," or the ability to change.

Medical research suggests that aerobic exercise can decrease cognitive impairment and reduce the risk of dementia. In fact, some researchers have suggested that it's time to prescribe physical activity for patients *with* dementia to improve cognitive function and the ability to perform activities of daily living such as eating, bathing, and getting to the toilet. So, forget about those video brain games: get up and move.

Enhanced Insulin Sensitivity

Glucose fuels almost every cell in the body, and insulin gets that glucose into cells. Some people develop what is called insulin resistance when the cells stop effectively utilizing insulin, requiring the beta cells of the pancreas to produce more and more insulin to get the same effects. This condition eventually leads to type 2 diabetes. Exercise can keep this at bay. In fact, a single bout of physical activity can lower blood glucose for at least two hours and as long as 72 hours.

But enhanced insulin sensitivity is not only important to lower glucose. Insulin resistance is linked to amyloid beta plaque formation, a feature of Alzheimer's disease. In addition, insulin-resistant individuals are at a greatly increased risk of developing certain forms of cancer. Even the American Cancer Society recommends physical activity to reduce cancer risk by maintaining a healthy weight and reducing insulin resistance. A large review found a 25% average reduction in risk of developing cancer among physically active women as compared to the least active women.

Longer, Healthier Life

Regular physical activity also decreases the risk of developing heart disease and stroke, even in the absence of weight loss. This is accomplished by reducing blood pressure, artery stiffness, visceral fat, and inflammation. Realize that some movement is better than no movement. One large study classified 400,000 men and women into five activity levels ranging from inactive to very high activity. Compared to the inactive group, those averaging just fifteen minutes a day had a three-year longer life expectancy.

Build Strong Bones

As we age, we lose bone mass. Exercise, especially aerobic impact and resistance exercise, helps to retain and even rebuild bone mass. Lifting weights isn't just to build muscles; weight-resistance exercise can prevent risk of bone fracture later in life. Of course, adequate protein, calcium, and vitamin D are also important for bone health.

Burns More Fat

When I run in the neighborhood, people remark, "Boy, you must love to run." Often my response is, "No, I love to eat." Active individuals have less body fat and more muscle mass, which results in a significantly higher resting metabolic rate, probably around 100 calories or more throughout the day. Add to that the calories burned during exercise and you can see that active people can burn significantly more calories than sedentary individuals.

While most adults tend to gain about a pound a year on the scale, the changes in body composition are more dramatic. That's because we tend to lose muscle and replace it with twice as much fat. If you start exercising and you don't see much change in the scale, don't give up. Muscles weigh more than fat, but they take up less space. As you lose body fat and add muscle, you'll soon see a positive change in the way your clothes fit.

Weight Maintenance

If you lose weight but stay inactive, there's a good chance that the weight is going to come right back on. That's because the number of calories we need is a factor of how much we weigh: the less we weigh, the fewer the calories we need to maintain that body size.

Losing about 10% of our body weight can result in a reduction in need of about 200 calories. For example, a 200-pound sedentary woman needs approximately 2600 calories to maintain her weight. Once she loses 20 pounds, she needs just 2400 calories. Obviously, weight maintenance will be much easier if she adds in another 200 calories worth of movement. Therefore, activity is the key to preventing such a major drop in metabolism when we lose weight.

Minimize Muscle Loss

While the goal during weight loss is to lose 100% fat, some muscle is always lost, too. Adding exercise can minimize muscle loss. In one study, healthy but overweight men were randomly placed into a control group or into one of three weight-loss groups that each lost about 20 pounds over a 12-week period. Those making only dietary changes lost 31% of that weight as muscle. Those combining diet with aerobic exercise three times a week lost 22% as muscle. The muscle loss was just 3% in the diet plus aerobic and strength-training group.

In another study, overweight men and women were divided into two groups that ate 25% fewer calories than they needed for six months. The first group reduced only their calories, while the second combined a calorie cut with additional exercise to create the same 25% calorie deficit. While those only cutting their calories initially lost more weight (and more muscle), after six months the weight loss was similar. Because those in the diet-only group lost more muscle mass, they needed 350 calories less per day to maintain their weight than those who exercised. So, clearly staying active to minimize muscle loss is critical if you want to keep off the weight lost and be able to eat more.

Appetite Control

Exercise, especially high-intensity exercise, helps control one's appetite. Unfortunately, some people overcompensate by eating more calories than they burn. I often see people at the gym who pedal slowly for 20 minutes while talking on the phone and then slip into the smoothie shop next door and order a 500-calorie drink. Interestingly, Dr. Wansink's research indicated that just *reading* about physical activity leads people to compensate by serving themselves more snacks. Though not statistically significant, when the physical activity was described as tiring rather than fun, snack consumption increased. That's another reason to focus on adding movements that you enjoy and think of as fun.

Better Sleep Quality

People who are physically active report sleeping better, even when the number of hours slept are the same. Inactive individuals often find themselves in a vicious cycle of not sleeping well and then not wanting to exercise the next day because they're tired. But, not exercising then further decreases sleep quality.

SIX SIMPLE STEPS FOR MOVING MORE

Ready to get moving? Here are six simple steps for incorporating more activity into your life:

Step 1: Consider the guidelines
Step 2: Make movements fun
Step 3: Find a way to fit it in
Step 4: Ramp it up
Step 5: Use it or lose it
Step 6: Sit less

Step 1: Consider the Guidelines

So we're both on the same page, let's take a look at the movement recommendations from the American College of Sports Medicine (ACSM). Please don't get overwhelmed, however. Once you review the other four steps for moving more, you'll realize how doable these recommendations are.

American College of Sports Medicine movement recommendations include:

- **Aerobic:** At least 150 minutes of moderate-intensity exercise each week (at least 30 minutes of moderate-intensity exercise five days a week) or 75 minutes vigorous-intensity exercise (20+ minutes three days a week).

- **Resistance:** Twice weekly resistance exercises to improve strength in each of the eight major muscle groups (shoulders, arms, back, abdomen, chest, butt, thighs, and calves). This involves doing 8–12 repetitions of a single movement (called a set), resting 2–3 minutes, and then repeating the set for a total of 2–4 times. Because resistance workouts break down the body (before building it back up stronger), a rest of 2–3 days between training sessions is recommended.

- **Flexibility:** Stretching muscles 2–3 days a week improves range of motion. Hold each stretch for 10–30 seconds and repeat 2–4 times for a total stretch time of 60 seconds per stretch. Stretches are most effective when muscle is warm, such as after a warm-up or exercise.

Step 2: Make Movements Fun

Ask anyone who has been exercising regularly for many years, and my guess is that they think what they do is fun. Stuart Brown, the psychiatrist who wrote *Play: How It Shapes the Brain, Opens the Imagination and Invigorates the Soul*, suggests that either we find time to play, or we'll find ourselves in a life without joy. He also says that the opposite of play isn't work but depression.

If you're not already moving on a regular basis, think about what you can do that would be so much fun you'd want to do it often. For me, it's tap dancing. I took it up in my early 20s, and, I've been tapping ever since. I plan to be tapping well into my 80s. I'm already the oldest student in my weekly class. In fact, one of the reasons I run is so I can keep up with all the younger tap students. At the end of this chapter is a list of 100+ fun ideas for moving more.

Step 3: Find a Way to Fit It In

At first glance, fitting in the ACSM exercise guidelines might sound like a lot of work, but it doesn't have to be. Here are some tips to fit movement into your busy day:

- **Take the short cut:** Did you notice that if you practice more intense movement, you can finish your workout in just 75 minutes a week (versus 150 minutes of moderate activity)? That's a savings of over an hour a week.

- **Break it up:** The ACSM specifies that the day's aerobic portion can be done at one time or in greater than 10-minute spurts, but even smaller spurts count. With adults in the Framingham Heart

Study, those accruing physical activity in short bouts of less than 10 minutes decreased their risk of a heart attack. Total moderate-to-vigorous activity was significantly associated with higher HDL and lower triglyceride levels, BMI, and waist circumference. So run the dog for 10 minutes in the morning, then join the neighborhood teenagers for an intense 10 minutes of basketball after work. Done!

- **Break it up further:** Some benefits can be obtained just one minute at a time. According to new research of 6,000 adults, an active lifestyle (as opposed to structured exercise) may be just as beneficial to staying healthy. That means counting even those little 1–2 minute moderate-intensity increments as part of the 30-minute requirement. So when you need a break at work, do a few simple exercises such as jumping jacks, sit-ups, and push-ups. Or just march in place.

- **Have a working-out lunch or meeting:** Instead of a working business lunch or a business discussion over drinks, opt to meet at the gym or on a walking path instead.

- **Go double duty:** Combine movement with something else you normally do. For example, run the treadmill while watching the news, read your favorite book only when you're on the exercise bike, and do squats every night while brushing your teeth. Do some pushups in the morning, an ab workout during TV commercials, and add some wall sits while cooking dinner (sit against the wall in the same position as if you had a chair).

- **Combine it all together:** Back in the 90s, I developed Dr. Jo®'s Hotel Room Workout for my book, *How to Stay Healthy & Fit on the Road.* The full-body workout involves alternating between one-minute intervals of aerobic exercise (such as jumping rope, jogging, or marching in place) with a set of resistance exercises using your body weight, hand weights, or exercise resistance bands. Just ten sets of each add up to a vigorous twenty-minute workout.

- **It doesn't have to be vigorous:** While vigorous movement has some additional benefits, even low levels of exercise on a regular basis can extend your life, decrease your weight, prevent major killer diseases, improve brain function, and give you more energy. Even a brief 10–20-minute walk can lower the glycemic effect of a meal, especially for individuals with type 2 diabetes.

- **Something is better than nothing:** Even if you don't have time for the full amount recommended, do something. More than 400,000 men and women participated in a standard medical screening program. Compared to the inactive group, those in the low-volume activity group who averaged 15 minutes a day had a 14% reduced risk of death from any cause; every additional 15 minutes of daily exercise further reduced all-cause mortality by 4%.

- **Make it part of your daily routine:** Trying to fit in a full-body flexibility workout 2–3 times a week doesn't work for me. We talked earlier about the benefits of having a healthy night-time ritual. For the past 20 years, I've made stretching part of my nighttime routine: just three to four stretches every night keeps me limber. Try adding stretches into your recovery breaks throughout the workday. Just take a brief walk to warm up those muscles before stretching.

- **Set your schedule:** Rest periods are recommended between workouts, so instead of being a weekend warrior, spread your movements through the week. For example, try an intense aerobic workout on Monday, Wednesday, and Friday, and do resistance workouts on Tuesday and Thursday.

- **Find a routine you can live with:** Instead of alternating between periods of working out every day for two hours, then doing nothing for weeks (or longer), find a level you can keep up long term.

- **Find a time that works for you:** What's the best time of the day to workout? Whatever time works best for you. If things tend to get in your way as the day goes on, work out first thing in the morning. Some find working out in the middle of the day makes them more productive in the afternoon. Evening workouts are good, too, unless the adrenaline rush prevents you from falling asleep.

- **Set a goal:** Sign up for a co-ed soccer league, a 5K run, or a fund-raising bike ride. A goal is a good way to stay motivated.

- **Have a back-up plan:** I have a friend who used to swim during his lunch hour, but when he developed bursitis in his shoulder, he stopped exercising completely because swimming was the only exercise he ever did. Your body will be healthier and stronger if you cross-train with more than one type of activity. And, you'll be more likely to stay in shape because you can be flexible. No pool? Go for a walk or run. Treadmill broken? Do Dr. Jo's Hotel Room Workout. What's your Plan B?

Step 4: Ramp It Up

Did you know that you burn the same number of calories whether you walk a mile or run a mile? A 150-pound person burns about 100 calories per mile. And, burning the same number of calories, at any intensity level, produces similar risk reductions in blood pressure and cholesterol levels, risk for diabetes mellitus, and possibly coronary heart disease.

That said, running may be better than walking for a couple of reasons. For one, runners can cover more miles in the same amount of time. So, while a walker can cover about four miles in an hour, a runner might be able to run eight, resulting in burning twice as many calories in that hour. But what if the runner stops at 30 minutes, covering the same four miles? Again, he'd burn 400 calories on the walk, but even if he sat down for the remaining 30 minutes, he'd still burn more calories than the walker in that hour.

The National Runners' and Walkers' Health Study, a 6.2-year follow-up study, found that walkers tended to burn fewer calories than runners throughout the day, and the walkers were significantly heavier than runners. Over six years, runners maintained their body weight and waistlines far better than walkers, even though runners tended to cut back more on their running (as measured by calories burned) than the walkers did. This was particularly noticeable among participants over 55 years of age.

Running might also help to curb appetite. In one study of women walkers and runners, participants worked out for 60 minutes and then were provided a meal to eat ad libitum. Not surprisingly, the runners ate more than the walkers. But, in total, the runners burned 200 calories *more than they ate*, while walkers ate 50 calories more than they burned.

Therefore, high-intensity vigorous activity might be more effective in managing weight than moderate-intensity exercise. In a random sample of more than 4,000 adults, only high-intensity physical activity was related to lower BMI. And the activity didn't have to be long. According to the study, every daily minute of high-intensity activity reduced the risk of obesity by 5% in women and by 2% in men. Each daily minute of high-intensity activity offsets the calorie equivalent of about half a pound. This means someone who regularly adds a minute of higher intensity activity each day will weigh nearly half a pound less than a person of similar height who is not as active.

That's probably because high-intensity movement builds more muscle mass. Take, for example, this small study of untrained and overfat women who were randomly assigned to either a high-intensity or low-intensity exercise group. They were instructed to make no diet or activity changes except to add exercise four times a week that burned 300 calories. Each lost about five pounds of fat. They both also added muscle, but the high-intensity group gained more than twice as much. Fat loss is a function of calories burned, but muscle increase is a factor of exercise intensity. And, remember, more muscle mass means burning more calories, so you can eat more.

Step 5: Use It or Lose It

With 1–2% of our body breaking down every day, it's important to practice intentional movement every two to three days to reap its continued benefits. After just three days of reduced physical activity, both post-meal glucose and insulin secretion increased. In as little as one to two weeks without exercise, many negative physiological changes occur. This can be detected in heart-rate variability, blood lipoproteins, glucose tolerance, insulin sensitivity, body composition, and inflammatory markers. The American Heart Association points out that with just five weeks of inactivity, you can lose 50% of your fitness ability.

Step 6: Sit Less

Even if you're getting in the recommended 30–60 minutes of exercise every day, what are you doing the other 23 hours? Chances are, you're sitting a lot. Research indicates we sit an average of nearly 8 hours a day, and interestingly, even exercisers tend to sit just as much. One study fitted 84 men and women with special shorts to measure activity in their thigh muscles and discovered virtually no difference in how much time people spent being couch potatoes comparing their exercise days with their non-exercise days.

So be honest with yourself: how much are you sitting? Just as people tend to underreport what they eat, they tend to over report how much they move. In one study, 1,751 adults wore an accelerometer (a device that tracks movement) for seven consecutive days and completed activity logs. On average, men and women reported more than two hours less sedentary time compared with what the accelerometer tracked. And although men reported 47% more moderate to vigorous physical activity compared with women, the tools measured no differences.

What's the big deal? There's a volume of research from countries all over the world that indicate the more you sit, the greater your risk of heart disease, diabetes, and death from all causes, especially when sitting ten or more hours. Sitting for long periods of time is associated with elevated blood pressure, glucose, triglycerides, and insulin. One study (using micro sensors worn under the clothes that measured movements every half second) found that leaner sedentary individuals are standing or moving around for about two and a half hours longer per day than obese participants. Workers who sit for long periods of time at their desk (measured objectively with a sitting pad) were nine times more likely to be overweight than those with lower sitting times.

More than two hours of TV viewing a day was also associated with a higher risk of overweight and obesity in both men and women. Some of this association may also be because sedentary people or those who watch a lot of TV tend to consume more fat and calories (especially in the evening) and less fiber. They also tend to eat less fruit and vegetables and eat more calorie-dense snacks, drinks, and fast food. The good news is that even if your job requires a lot of sitting, moderate to vigorous physical activity appears to reduce the hazardous association between sitting and death.

HOW TO DECREASE SEDENTARY TIME

Because excess sitting can lead to increases in weight along with a decrease in energy and health, it's important to incorporate strategies such as these:

- **Cut your commute:** Longer commutes are associated with less physical activity, lower cardiorespiratory fitness, and more body fat.

- **Stand up or sit on a large inflatable therapy ball:** A 150-pound person burns around 100 calories an hour sitting and 135 calories an hour standing, with sitting on a therapy ball somewhere in between. It doesn't sound like much, but every calorie adds up over the hours.

- **Break up your sedentary time:** An Australian study found that regardless of how long they were sedentary or participated in moderate- to-vigorous-intensity activity, increased breaks in sedentary time (measured with an accelerometer) were associated with lower two-hour glucose levels, triglycerides, waist circumference, and BMI. Think about it: if you were to get up and move just four minutes during every waking hour, you'd shave an hour off your total sitting time.

- **Use a pedometer:** Step-counting devices can provide motivation to get up and move to reach a goal of about 10,000 steps a day. You can use a simple $10 pedometer or choose a more advanced one (such as the Fitbit or Nike JawBone) in the $100 range.

- **Fidget more:** You don't just burn calories while working out. Fidgeting and other small movements (referred to as non-exercise activity thermogenesis or NEAT) burns calories, too. So tap your foot to the music and get up and stretch periodically.

- **Work on a treadmill:** There are now standing desks and treadmill and stationary-bike stations that allow you to get your work done while burning a few more calories. One study with sedentary obese individuals found sitting in an office chair burned 72 calories per hour, while walking and working on a slow-moving treadmill (1.1 mph) burned 191 calories, a difference of 119 calories per hour. With everything else held constant, working at a treadmill desk just one hour per workday could potentially lead to a weight loss of nearly ten pounds in a year.

- **Move every chance you get:** Pace the house or do some light dusting while talking on the phone. Walk, bike, or skate wherever you need to go. Stand up during a meeting. Take the stairs instead of the elevator. Walk to a colleague's desk instead of picking up the phone or park a bit farther at the mall or office to add a few more steps. Do sit-ups or push-ups during TV commercials. Walk the kids to school. Go for an evening walk instead of watching TV. At the office, use the rest room on another floor. Walk briskly while doing errands.

100+ FUN IDEAS FOR MOVING MORE

Forget about getting bored at the gym. There are so many other fun ways to move:

- **Go on active vacations:** People frequently talk about vacations in terms of how many pounds they gained, as if every fun vacation has to include a few extra pounds. It does not! Fun and weight gain need not go together. To balance out those extra vacation treats, take vacations that include daily play including hikes, bike rides, snorkeling, horseback riding, mountain climbing, and more.

- **Play ball:** Join a sports team such as baseball, basketball, softball, football, flag football, soccer, water polo, volleyball, kickball, lacrosse, rugby, or even ping-pong. You might even be able to find an organized quidditch team (yes, sort of like what Harry Potter played) in your area. Check out the International Quidditch Association at www.iquaquidditch.com.

- **Find a rink:** Go ice skating or find a hockey or broom-hockey team (you don sneakers instead of skates).

- **Kick it up a notch:** Find an aerobic-dance, jazzercise, Zumba, cardio-dance, or kickboxing class. In your area, you might even find hoola-hoop classes, RipSurferX (an aerobics class that simulates surfing), or pound rock out workouts (beating the floor with a pair of weighted drumsticks).

- **Get strong with slow movements:** Try yoga, Pilates, Tai Chi, qigong, or Nia (a cool blend of yoga, martial arts, and dance).

- **Take a dance class:** If you enjoy watching the TV shows "Dancing with the Stars" or "So You Think You can Dance," search for a dance class at your local dance studio, community center, or community college. Try traditional ballet, jazz, tap, or hip hop. There's also ballroom (including waltz, fox trot, rhumba, East-Coast and West-Coast swing), Latin (salsa, bachata, merengue, samba), dances from other time periods (Charleston and Lindy), country western, tango, hustle, nightclub two-step, and line dancing.

- **Go exotic:** Try pole dance, ribbon dance, belly dance, or Bollywood dance classes. One of my readers wrote, "I signed up for belly dancing classes. My boys think it's cool, my daughter thinks I'm crazy, and my husband bought me a coin belt."

- **Get wet:** You can swim laps (even underwater), tread water, or go aqua walking wearing sneakers and weights around your middle, or find a water-aerobics class.

- **Hit the open water:** I'm no Bethany Hamilton. Standing on my nine-foot foam-top surfboard on two-foot Florida waves is nothing like surfing the 20-foot Pipeline in Hawaii, but I'm still surfing, and I didn't start till my 50s. Maybe it's time for you to hit the open water and surf, canoe, kayak, row, paddleboard (SUP), wind surf, or snorkel. Or, have fun jumping from rock to rock in a shallow stream.

- **Practice martial arts:** The most common ones are judo, karate, and Taekwondo, but there's also aikido (a defensive Japanese martial arts where you redirect the force of the attack), Krav Maga (a self-defense system developed for the military in Israel) or capoeira (a Brazilian martial arts done with song and dance).

- **Play with the kids (or just act like one):** You'll feel younger when you hop, skip, jump, or do jumping jacks. Do cart wheels and summersaults. Try a pogo stick, skateboard, or a weighted hula hoop. Play jump rope, Chinese jump rope, double dutch, or hopscotch. Shoot some hoops, play catch, or take a gymnastics class.

- **Use your imagination:** One time we forgot the ball when we went to the pool, then we found out it's a hoot to play keep away with an *imaginary* ball. Make-believe jump rope is even harder than the real thing because you never trip on the rope.

- **Cardio clean:** I met a woman who told me, "With four kids, I really don't have any time to myself and no time to go to the gym, so I came up with this idea of turning my housecleaning chore into something fun." She bought an apron from the hardware store to hold all her tools: sprays, rags, and such. Then, she turned up the stereo real loud and cleaned everything from top to bottom in a clockwise direction. "I've discovered that the faster the music, the faster I can clean the house."

- **Take a few laps:** Bike, run, rollerblade, or roller skate around the block or around town.

- **Go extreme (with your doctor's permission):** More intense workouts include boxing, P90X, CrossFit, boot camps, ViPR, or agility workouts (it's not just for dogs anymore).

- **Sweat it out:** Go disco dancing or take the stairs at the office just for the fun of it.

- **Go outside:** Take a brisk walk, go mountain or rock climbing, or play on the outdoor gym. Golf (where you can ditch the cart) or take up orienting (a compass-based race in the woods). Try Frisbee® or disc golf; there are about 3,000 parks in the U.S where you count how many throws it takes to get a Frisbee® from hole to hole (a mesh basket sitting up on a pole).

- **Get dirty:** If this suits you, there are now plenty of running races, bike rides, and obstacle course races in the mud (search for mud runs and rides on the internet).

- **Hit the trails:** Opt for hiking, trail running, trail bike riding, horseback riding, snowshoeing, and cross-country skiing. Check out your city or county parks. There are plenty of trails at U.S. national or state parks and national parks of Canada.

- **Head to the slopes:** Go skiing, snowboarding, or tubing.

- **Play on the court:** Choose from tennis, handball, racquetball, squash, or even pickleball.

- **Use obstacles to your advantage:** Parcour, a sport in many urban settings, is described as the fastest way to get from A to B and involves running, jumping, and climbing things that get in your way.

- **Walk with a purpose:** Take your next walk with a predetermined purpose such as checking out the landscaping, looking for birds or animals, or practicing a speech. If you're planning a move, walking is a good way to explore potential neighborhoods.

- **Walk somewhere different:** Looking for a scenic and safe place to walk, especially while away from home? Check out American Volkssport Association (AVA). The AVA network consists of hundreds of clubs that organize walking events. They also offer marked or mapped routes to walk on your own. Go to www.ava. org and click on the "Find Walking Events" link to find walks near you or where you're heading.

- **Stay home:** Try a Wii workout or buy an indo board to practice surfing in your living room. One of my clients lost over 70 pounds, not so much by changing what she ate, but by turning on the radio after dinner and dancing with the kids. Everyone looked forward to Dance Night.

- **Find a friend:** Have you ever wanted to get into an activity but didn't know how to get started or didn't want to go alone? Then, check out www.meetup.com. While some people use meetup. com to find dates or groups involved in sedentary activities such as book clubs or networking groups, it's also a free place to find people that enjoy the same things that you like to do like dancing, kayaking, hiking, and more.

- **Get lost in a movie:** My friend, Janet, hadn't exercised regularly in her 50+ years until she found a fitness center that offered a cardio movie theatre where you can plug in a movie while working out on aerobic equipment. Like Janet, you just might find yourself working out longer as you get caught up in the movie. No such fitness center near you? Park your exercise bike or treadmill in front of your TV at home and pop in a movie.

For additional ideas, check out the Wall Street Journal's weekly column, "What's Your Workout?" which features the exercise routines of business execs who recognize that movement is critical to their success.

13

Refueling Around Movement

If your movement routine includes gardening, a slow stroll, or any other exercise that barely gets your heart rate up, you don't need to eat any different than what was already suggested. On the other hand, if you're active (or plan to be) it helps to tweak your eating habits before, during, and after workouts. Doing so can enhance your performance, body composition, and post-workout recovery for these four reasons:

- **Active individuals burn more calories:** To maximize training effects, these additional calories are best provided by eating more often throughout the day (every three to four hours).

- **Building muscle is a two-step process:** First, you exercise to break down the muscle, and then you rebuild it stronger. In order to rebuild muscle, you need protein plus adequate calories to do the rebuilding.

- **Active muscles burn a greater percent of glucose:** As activity intensity increases, the body shifts from a 50/50 glucose-fat ratio to a fuel mix that's more concentrated in glucose. This requires a plan to maintain blood glucose levels and maximize glycogen stores.

- **It's important to replace our sweat losses:** Because even slight dehydration can affect performance, we need to start out hydrated and continue to drink fluids during and after exercise to replace losses.

Les was an avid exerciser. He worked out nearly every morning for an hour, including both aerobic and resistance exercises. While he said he felt good during the workouts, he recently felt his energy waning and his thinking was getting more "fuzzy" and blamed it on his age. As it turned out, his age wasn't the reason. While he was doing the work necessary to get stronger, he wasn't refueling effectively before, during, or after his workouts.

Even if you do all the right body work, you're not going to build a strong, lean body if you don't provide the body with the raw materials it needs to make the changes. Not refueling will also affect your energy and performance, too. That's a shame because many people (like Celine from Chapter 6 with complaints of cellulite) do the work but don't get all the benefits they should be getting.

PRE-WORKOUT FUELING

The most important pre-workout consideration is to ensure that glucose and glycogen stores are adequate to meet your impending workout needs. This includes both liver glycogen and muscle glycogen.

Because exercising muscles obtain their glucose needs primarily from muscle glycogen, you'll perform better, longer, and faster on a full reserve of muscle glycogen. As long as you've been eating the recommended amounts of carbohydrate on a regular basis, your muscle glycogen levels are adequate to fuel moderate activity. Running out of glycogen contributes to muscle fatigue even during mild exercise, but it's even more noticeable during longer events. One study found that participants sustained aerobic exertion for 90 minutes on a low-carb, high-fat diet, 120 minutes on a normal diet, and 240 minutes with a high-carb diet. Realize that without adequate muscle glycogen stores, the muscles will draw the glucose fuel from the bloodstream, dropping levels dangerously low.

Active individuals need more calories, so it's best to fuel the body by eating every three to four hours. This allows for consistent fuel for the brain and red blood cells, which run on either the glucose from a previous meal or snack or the glucose that is stored in liver glycogen. If you start to exercise when your liver glycogen is in a depleted state, your brain and red blood cells will continue to draw glucose from the bloodstream, requiring an increasing amount of muscle to be broken down and converted to glucose, and that's not good. Remember, even if your muscle glycogen stores are full, it cannot leave the muscles, so it's not available to fuel the brain.

If you plan on working out for an hour (or less), and you just ate one to two hours ago, there's no need to have a pre-workout snack. For a two-hour workout, eat no more than one hour before. In other words, if by the time you finish your exercise, it will be longer than three hours since you last ate, it's critical to eat something before exercising.

To Eat or Not to Eat Before Morning Exercise

Les didn't eat anything before his morning workout because he'd heard that *not* eating before exercise burns *more fat*. And, because he didn't have an appetite after working out, he waited until he got into work several hours later to slip into the cafeteria and eat something small like a bowl of oatmeal. Holding off breakfast until midmorning was contributing to his lack of energy.

Because the body is somewhat capable of adjusting to whatever fuel is available, there is some truth that we burn more fat if we workout before breakfast. But that's only half the story. When we exercise, we need two sources of glucose. First, the active muscles need glucose because aerobic workouts require a greater percentage of glucose as fuel. Again, if you've been eating carbs on a regular basis, your muscle glycogen should be adequate to fuel this activity. If you haven't been eating carbs, you'll be training in a low-glycogen state. This is associated with an increasing amount of stress hormones being released.

Second, we need glucose for the brain and red blood cells. While we slept, the body used nearly all our liver glycogen to meet our glucose needs. By the time we wake up in the morning, most of the glucose needed is being provided from the breakdown of protein. The longer you go without eating, the more muscle mass your body needs to break down (and, let's face it, the more exercise you'll need to do to replace it).

If you don't eat carbs before working out, the body has no choice but to burn more fat. But in order to meet its basic glucose needs, this will also require the body to break down more lean muscle mass. Overtime, this loss of muscle mass will lower your metabolic rate. So eat something, even if it's small, before your morning workout. If you're watching your weight, remember that breakfast eaters tend to burn more calories both during exercise and after.

What to Eat Before Exercise

Pre-exercise snacks or meals improve performance when they consist of mostly carbohydrates to maintain blood glucose and maximize glycogen stores, and possibly some protein. As mentioned earlier, it's a good idea to take in 20–30g of protein before or right after exercise. Because it takes two to three hours for proteins from foods to enter the bloodstream, you might want to have some of it before working out (to counter the net loss of muscle protein during exercise). You can also wait and have the protein after (for rebuilding purposes).

The pre-workout foods need to be well tolerated. These tend to be foods that are relatively low in fat and fiber that leave your stomach quickly and do not cause GI upset. Caution with caffeine: a small amount of caffeine (about 100mg or a short cup of coffee) 10–40 minutes before exercise can improve mental focus, alertness, and may help the muscles to use more fat as a fuel, which delays depletion of muscle glycogen. On the other hand, caffeine may also cause GI upset and temporarily increase urine flow. To start off your activity well hydrated, drink 8–16oz of water just before your workout and adjust to factors including heat, humidity, and exercise intensity.

The size of a pre-workout snack is determined by the length of the activity. For activities lasting an hour or less, start with about 100 calories. This may include a cup of yogurt or milk, half a toasted English muffin with peanut butter, banana, or 100-calorie snack bar. A larger snack of 200–300 calories (or even a full meal) might be more appropriate when working out longer than an hour. Appendix H has suggestions for other 100- to 300-calorie snacks.

WORKOUT FUEL

During a workout, your muscles burn more carbohydrates than they do at rest, especially as the intensity increases. In addition, because you're sweating, your fluid and electrolyte needs increase. Therefore, depending on exercise duration, you may need to refuel during your workout.

Activities Less Than One Hour

If you ate a small snack or meal before working out, and you're planning on eating a meal shortly after, there's no need for carbs or protein during a workout of an hour or less. Just drink water to replace your sweat loss. If you're exercising first thing in the morning when glycogen stores are low (and don't feel like eating breakfast first), consume a sports drink with carbohydrates during this shorter activity to keep your blood glucose levels in the normal range. In addition, athletes participating in intense stop-and-go activities such as soccer or football might also benefit from carbohydrates during these activities, even if it's less than an hour of exercise.

Activities Lasting Longer Than One Hour

It's called bonking, crashing, or hitting the wall. When athletes run out of glycogen, they quickly loose speed as their blood glucose falls and the body burns more protein to bring it back up. To provide this constant glucose need, it's a good idea to eat or drink a source of carbohydrate when exercising continuously for longer than an hour. Consider this study with endurance cyclists. They were able to bike for three hours with a flavored water solution (placebo). But, drinking a glucose solution allowed them to cycle for four hours by allowing the muscles to burn the glucose from the drink, thereby sparing some of the muscle glycogen.

Keep in mind that trained endurance athletes generally have much larger glycogen stores than most of us. If you are participating in activities longer than an hour, it's a good idea to eat or drink carbs *before* you're feeling hungry or tired (which may be a sign of glycogen depletion), which is usually 30–60 minutes after the start of exercise; then, eat at frequent intervals, like every 15 minutes. Choose foods and drinks that are easy on your stomach (it's different for different people) such as a fluid-replacement beverage. For most of us, there's no need to add protein during exercise; the protein you eat throughout the day will be adequate.

Fluid Replacement Beverages

Consuming 30–60 g of carbohydrates per hour will help you maintain normal blood glucose levels, so you can work out longer and harder and keep your energy up. The recommendation is based on the fact that, due to saturation of what the intestinal tract can transport, athletes can only metabolize a certain amount of carbohydrate at a time. Taking in more carbs won't increase your performance and may cause you problems if the drink is sitting in the GI tract.

Because fluid losses due to sweat also need to be replaced, the easiest way to replenish your carbs is with a sports drink containing 6–8% carbohydrates, such as Gatorade or Powerade, which is most quickly absorbed into your bloodstream. These drinks contain 14g of carbohydrate per 8 fluid ounces, so drinking about 8–16 fluid ounces every 10–15 minutes provide both the glucose and the fluid you need. Looking on the label, you'll notice that many of these drinks contain more than one type of sugar. That's intentional, because better utilization occurs when the carbohydrate consists of two or more sugars (sucrose, fructose, glucose, maltodextrins), rather than just one. Some athletes prefer solid forms of carbohydrates such as gels, shots, or bars, and then drink just plain water. Other people prefer low-fat foods such as raisins, bananas, pretzels, or candy including hard candies, Twizzlers, jelly beans, or gummy bears. Both solid and liquid forms of glucose are equally effective in maintaining normal glucose levels and improving performance; added protein and fat only delay gastric emptying.

Sodas, fruit juices, and energy drinks are *not* recommended during exercise because they contain a higher concentration of carbohydrate, which slows down emptying time in the stomach. Long after you drink it, they are still sitting in your stomach causing GI upset and not in your blood stream where it's needed.

Low- or no-calorie electrolyte beverages are also not recommended for long activities because they contain little or no glucose, and glucose replacement is just as important as fluid replacement. I've often heard people say they choose these no- or low-calorie electrolyte beverages for the first hour (to save calories), and then switch to a 6% carbohydrate sports drink afterwards. You'll maintain glucose levels and perform better if you drink the 6% drink throughout the entire event. Think about it: when you run faster and longer with the recommended drinks, you'll burn more calories.

What Workout Intensity Burns More Fat?

We are always burning an ever-changing combination of fuel. The more intense the aerobic exercise is, the more glucose that's burned by the muscle:

- **Low-intensity:** 10–15% glucose + 85–90% fat
- **Moderate intensity:** 50–60% glucose + 40–50% fat
- **High-intensity:** 70–80% glucose + 20–30% fat
- **All-out sprint:** 100% glucose

If your goal is to lose weight, it's easy to think that because low-intensity exercise burns a higher percentage of fat it's the better choice to burn more body fat. But, it's not. To lose body fat, you need to focus on creating a calorie deficit by burning more calories than you eat. While a greater *percentage* of fat is burned during low-intensity exercise, *more calories* are burned during high-intensity exercise. To illustrate, let's estimate calorie burn over a one-hour workout using a 160-pound person as an example:

- **Low intensity:** A brisk walk (4 miles per hour) for 60 minutes burns 438 calories. Assuming a 15% glycogen/85% fat ratio, about 66 calories is from glycogen and 372 calories from fat.

- **Moderate intensity:** Running 6 miles an hour would burn 715 calories in one hour. At a 50/50 fuel ratio, that works out to be 358 calories from each glycogen and fat.

- **High intensity:** Running 8.5 miles an hour burns about 898 calories in an hour. Because about 80% of the calories would come from glycogen, that's about 718 calories from glycogen and just 180 calories from fat.

So, find a workout you enjoy that burns the most calories for you. In the long run, that's what will help you decrease body fat. Consider which activity you enjoy and which level you can keep up for a long enough period of time to achieve your goals. If you can exercise at a moderate pace for an hour, but only fifteen minutes if the exercise is intense, you might opt for the more moderate pace to burn more calories.

POST-WORKOUT FUELING

As discussed in Chapter 7, athletic individuals manage energy best when they eat every three or four hours. Eating after a workout is not necessarily another eating opportunity because it often falls in line with the timing of a typical meal or a snack. Though depending on the length and intensity of the workout, the composition may need to be tweaked.

Low-intensity workouts burn very little glycogen, so no additional post-workout fuel is needed; the usual meal or snack (as we outlined previously) will suffice. If you exercise moderately just a few times a week, and you're already eating every three or four hours, you may not need to do anything differently than you normally would because there'll be many meals and snacks to refuel before the next workout.

If you work out five or more times a week, you have two workouts in a day, or a long workout, your post-workout nutrition needs are more critical. You'll need adequate carbohydrates to replenish your glycogen stores quickly, protein to provide the raw material to rebuild your muscles stronger, and fluid and electrolytes that are lost in sweat to be replaced.

Carbohydrates

At capacity, about 1% of muscle weight is glycogen. Therefore, the more muscle mass you have, the more glycogen you can store. A normal, lean athletic man would have roughly 300 g of glycogen. Because every gram of carbohydrate contains four calories, that's 1,200 calories' worth of muscle glycogen. You may have more or less.

Full glycogen stores allow you to workout harder and longer. So, it's important to use the post-workout fueling to replenish these stores. Glycogen stores can be replaced anytime, but you can *double* your glycogen stores if you eat carbohydrates within the first thirty minutes after exercise (versus waiting two hours after). If you have a sweet tooth, this might be the best time to eat your favorites. Carbohydrates with a high GI (such as bread, cereal, soda, candy, cookies, and the like) result in higher muscle glycogen levels 24 hours after a glycogen-depleting exercise compared with the same amount of low GI carbs.

If you're watching your weight, realize that there's no need to replace the total calories you've burned during your work out. Your aim should be to replace just the glycogen (not the fat) that was burned, so it's there for your next workout. So if mostly high-carbohydrate items are consumed following exercise, the amount of food needed to replenish the glycogen reserves is always far less than the energy expended during the exercise.

Aim for about 0.5g carbohydrate per pound of body weight. That's 75 g carbs for a 150-pound person and 100 g for a 200-pound athlete. Consume that amount within thirty minutes of completing your workout, then again every two hours for four to six hours. If your workout was intense, chances are you'll soon be hungry for more food, and the amounts should be easily achievable.

Protein

Building strong muscles is a two-step process. The exercise first breaks down muscle mass, then the body rebuilds the muscles stronger. While the body is constantly replacing the proteins that have broken down, when you eat protein around the time of either resistance or endurance exercise, the synergistic interaction results in a greater muscle mass than when just eating protein alone. If you don't eat protein after working out, you may have just wasted your time. Here's an analogy to consider. Building a home requires two things: building materials and a crew to do the work. If the crew shows up, but there's no building materials, you can't build a house. The same thing happens with exercise – if you do the work (exercise), but don't provide the body with the essential building materials (dietary protein), your body can't build the body stronger.

The best window of opportunity to have protein available for muscle building is within the first three hours after exercise. Because it takes a couple of hours to digest intact proteins from foods (such as meat, eggs, cheese, and soy beans), eat protein at the same time as the carbohydrates (within thirty minutes after you finish exercising) to double the amount of protein laid down as muscle. Aim for about 20–30g protein; more muscle synthesis does not occur with more protein. If you have very high protein needs, just continue to 20–30 g of protein at regular intervals of every three or four hours throughout the day.

If you don't have much of an appetite after an intense workout, drink a liquid protein. Not only do liquids quench thirst, these proteins enter the bloodstream faster than solid ones. While there are plenty of powdered proteins (whey, casein, egg, soy, and pea proteins) you can add to smoothies, the least expensive liquid protein is dairy milk. Chocolate milk is an effective recovery beverage because it has both carbohydrate and protein in the recommended

4:1 ratio similar to many commercial recovery beverages (one 8-fluid-ounce cup of chocolate milk contains 32 g of carbohydrate and 8g of protein). This protein-plus-carbohydrate combination has also been associated with reductions in markers of muscle damage and improved post-exercise recovery.

Milk is composed of two proteins (80% casein and 20% whey). Both proteins are rich sources of branched-chain amino acids (which enhance muscle protein synthesis), so you don't need to spend extra money on supplements. Of course, chocolate milk is not the only option. You could drink a glass of nonfat milk and add more carbohydrates in the form of a peanut butter sandwich or even brownies.

Remember Les, the man mentioned earlier in this chapter who was feeling fuzzy-headed after his workouts? Like him, if you're not eating anything before or immediately after workouts the body is not going to be able to do build the muscle you desire. It's not going to rebuild the glycogen stores that are necessary to get you through your next workout, either. Without those glycogen stores, you won't be able to work out as hard and as long as you could with that additional fuel. Insufficient fueling before or after work-outs not only leads to poor muscle building, as Les found out, the body and brain are left undernourished and feeling fuzzy-headed.

Fluid

As discussed earlier, 1% dehydration can affect energy and mood, while dehydration levels above 2% of your body weight can also affect performance. The best way to estimate your fluid loss from sweat loss is to weigh yourself (without clothes) both before and after exercise, as detailed below. If you're not around a scale, check the color of your urine: it should be clear. Yellow urine indicates dehydration, although certain medications and supplements can affect the color.

Jay was a 200-pound guy who biked long distances on the weekend. He was looking for a better fluid-replacement beverage because the rides were wiping him out for the rest of the weekend. I asked him to weigh himself without clothes both before and im-mediately after his long rides. It turns out that Jay was down nearly 10 pounds after his rides. Because each pound that is lost represents two cups of fluid, he had lost 20 cups of water. As it turned out, it wasn't the choice of the drink that caused his fatigue but the fact he wasn't drinking enough. From then on, Jay drank 16 ounces before starting a ride and then took a more methodical approach to rehydrating himself during the ride to make sure he stayed hydrated. For him, this added up to drinking about 12 ounces every 15 minutes.

Appendixes

Appendix A: Medical Causes of Fatigue
Appendix B: Preventing the Mid-Day Slump
Appendix C: What to Do When You're Crashing
Appendix D: Strategies to Lose Weight While Staying Energized
Appendix E: Breakfast Ideas
Appendix F: Lunch Ideas
Appendix G: Dinner Ideas
Appendix H: Snack Ideas

Appendix A: Medical Causes of Fatigue

If your energy is waning and you can't seem to bounce back, it's important to rule out medical issues by having a full medical exam by a physician. Fatigue can sometimes be a nonspecific symptom of a more serious problem. The following are the most common medical causes of fatigue:

- **Diabetes:** A group of diseases where the body can't use blood glucose normally, resulting in high blood glucose levels. It affects 9% of the U.S. population.

- **Hypothyroidism:** Low levels of thyroid hormones can lower your metabolic rate and make you feel more tired. It affects 1–2% of the population and is more common in women.

- **Depression:** If you're feeling sad and can't find pleasure in things you once enjoyed, you might be depressed. Tell your doctor or therapist.

- **Undiagnosed heart disease:** Fatigue can be a sign of heart trouble.

- **Insomnia:** A sleep disorder including difficulty falling asleep, staying awake much of the night, waking up early, or waking feeling unrefreshed.

- **Obstructive sleep apnea:** A condition where the airway collapses, cutting off breathing for ten seconds or more. Due to lack of oxygen, the body wakes itself up to start breathing again. Although one may not be fully aware of these frequent wakings, the result is extreme fatigue even with adequate time spent in bed.

- **Restless leg syndrome:** A disorder where unpleasant sensations in the legs cause a strong urge to move them, perhaps causing involuntary leg twitching or jerking, especially when trying to relax for sleep.

- **Narcolepsy:** A rare, chronic neurological disorder resulting in frequent "sleep attacks" (falling asleep instantly for several seconds to more than thirty minutes) during the day, even with a normal amount of sleep at night.

- **Infections:** Illnesses such as infectious mononucleosis, chronic sinus infections, and urinary tract infections can cause fatigue as the immune system directs energy to fight the cause of the infection.

- **Uncontrolled allergies:** Chronic symptoms such as a runny nose and fatigue are often easily treated and self-managed.

- **Medications:** Fatigue can also occur as a side effect of medications such as muscle relaxants, antibiotics, sedative-hypnotics (medications to reduce tension and bring on sleep), blood pressure medications, antidepressants, and antihistamines (even nonsedating ones).

- **Chronic fatigue syndrome:** A relatively rare condition in which fatigue lasts longer than six months along with four or more specific symptoms including muscle pain, headaches of a new type, pain in joints without swelling or redness, and a sore throat that is frequent or recurring.

- **Anemia:** A condition where the bloodstream can't transport as much oxygen to the rest of the body, noted by a deficiency of red blood cells or hemoglobin (a protein in red blood cells). The most common causes of anemia include low levels of iron, vitamin B12, and folate (or folic acid). Before you diagnose yourself and take supplements, it's important to consult your doctor for a blood test. Proper diagnosis is important in getting the right treatment. For example, taking a folate supplement may change the red blood cells to appear "cured" but mask irreversible, potentially severe damage to the nervous system caused by a B12 deficiency.

- **Vitamin D deficiency:** While it's been said that we only need fifteen minutes of exposure to our face, arms, and hands at least twice a week without sunscreen to get adequate vitamin D levels, the Institute of Medicine estimates that one third of adults are deficient; very low levels are associated with muscle weakness.

Appendix B: Preventing the Mid-Day Slump

If you frequently experience mid-afternoon lows, try to figure out what's happening, so you can prevent a repeat. Here are questions to ask yourself:

1.   **Am I getting enough of the right type of sleep?** A mid-afternoon dip is a feature of your circadian rhythm. Like the "low" we experience in the middle of the night that makes it difficult to stay awake, a similar low period occurs in the middle of the afternoon. The more sleep deprived we are, the more tired we feel in the middle of the afternoon. Solution: get adequate sleep on a consistent basis.

2.   **Am I dehydrated?** Even slight dehydration can affect your energy level, mood, and concentration. Check the color of your urine; it should be clear to very light. Solution: keep a water bottle with you at all times and sip throughout the day.

3.   **Did I eat breakfast today?** Breakfast is the most important meal of the day because it jump-starts your metabolism. When you skip breakfast, the body starts conserving energy for the crucial tasks of keeping you alive, leaving you feeling lethargic and fuzzy headed. The longer you go without eating, the more muscle protein is converted into glucose for the brain and red blood cells. Hungry for glucose, the body will overreact to the carbs eaten at the next meal (lunch), sending your blood glucose on a roller-coaster ride of highs and lows. Solution: eat breakfast every day.

4.   **Did I get enough fuel at lunch?** While a normal-sized meal should last 3–4 hours, a smaller meal will last only 2–3 hours. So, your energy drop at 3 p.m. could just signify the need to eat a snack. Solution: Learn to listen to your body and eat to refuel as necessary.

5.   **Have I eaten enough today?** Perhaps you ate breakfast and lunch, but the total calories are way less than the body needs. At some point during the day, the body will scream, "ENOUGH!!" and demand food NOW! You may not recognize this scream as hunger; it might present itself as low energy. Solution: spread out your food intake throughout the whole day rather than eating most of it in the evening.

6.   **Am I running on fuel or stimulants?** Caffeine doesn't fuel your body: it's a stimulant drug. Stress does the same thing to our body; it makes you feel alert. But neither can fuel the brain, so the body still responds as if you haven't eaten enough and leaves you crashing when these stimulants run out. Solution: Don't rely upon caffeine or stress to keep you alert. Eat on a regular basis.

7.   **Did I wait too long to fuel?** When you put off eating for too long, and your blood glucose starts to fall, the body switches to liver glycogen stores and possibly even muscles to fuel the body. This is good because it brings back up your glucose to normal levels. Unfortunately, because that low blood glucose also made you feel ravenous, chances are you will overeat at that next meal, sending your glucose levels on a roller-coaster ride and landing you at the very bottom shortly after lunch. Solution: Eat when you're feeling hungry; don't wait until you're ravenous or you'll likely overeat.

8.   **Did I eat high GI/GL?** Excessive amounts of fast-acting carbs (high GI) give you a short burst of quick energy, eventually leaving your glucose at rock bottom in just 1–2 hours (especially during the mid-afternoon low in the circadian rhythm). Solution: Slow-acting carbs (low GI) provide you with a steady source of energy without the crash. Instead of high-GI foods (such as sodas, sweets, processed cereal, and breads), reach for low-GI foods like less-processed whole grains, milk, oats, beans, and fresh fruit.

9.   **Did I eat too many carbs at lunch?** Carbohydrates are digested, absorbed, and cleared from the bloodstream within two hours after eating, returning blood glucose back to normal levels. The body's inability to do this is indicative of diabetes. Solution: there's no need to be on a low-carbohydrate diet (carbs fuel our brain, red blood cells, and exercising muscles), but it's important not to eat too many at one time. Some individuals (such as women and people over 50) seem to be more sensitive to high-carbo-hydrate meals at lunchtime and feel this dip just an hour or two afterwards.

10.   **Did I eat enough protein?** Protein not only builds muscle and helps us feel full longer, it also stabilizes blood glucose between meals. Solution: always eat 20–30 g of protein at each meal.

Appendix C: What to Do When You're Crashing

If it's too late and you're already feeling your energy wane, try these suggestions to instantly treat the midday slump:

- **Switch gears:** Rather than working on a project that requires a large amount of brain power, it helps to do more menial tasks at this time of the day.

- **Get up and move:** Take a brisk walk or run up a few flights of stairs. Jumping jacks will definitely wake you up.

- **Take a power nap:** Tell the boss you need to run a quick errand, then go out to the car and take a short powernap. A quick 10–30 minute nap is usually effective in relieving sleepiness.

- **Drink caffeine:** Research supports that a small dose (50–100 mg) does the trick (that's a very short cup of coffee; refer back to chapter 3 for more details). More is not better. If you're going to take a nap, too, have the caffeine first. Because caffeine takes 15–30 minutes to enter your bloodstream, it will be at its peak when you wake from your nap.

- **Have a snack:** If you start to crash mid-afternoon, and it feels like your blood glucose is dropping, don't put off eating. Eat a small, low-GI snack containing both carbs and protein such as milk, yogurt, or cheese and an apple. If you're already feeling like you've put off refueling for too long (especially if you're now feeling shaky and weak), focus on eating a higher-protein snack. That shaky feeling suggests the body is already increasing blood glucose levels by chiseling up body stores; protein will help stabilize the glucose, preventing another rebound. See Appendix H for some snack ideas.

Appendix D: Strategies to Lose Weight While Staying Energized

Energized individuals are more likely to lose fat weight than their sedentary, sluggish friends. Here are some tips to help you achieve your goals:

- **Energy first:** When you're feeling fat and fatigued, it's tempting to work on losing weight to regain your energy. But, that's backwards. When you focus on regaining your energy, you'll find yourself with the willpower to say no to your teasers and the innate desire to want to move more, all of which will promote weight loss.

- **Slow is best:** We all like to see the numbers on the scale descend rapidly, but remember a quick loss is indicative of a major decrease in glycogen stores and muscle mass (both are about 75% water content). Glycogen losses can decrease your physical activity endurance, while loss of muscles will further lower your metabolism, making it hard to keep the weight off. Aim for losing no more than a pound or two a week. Many people with successful weight loss kept it to just a quarter or half pound a week. The slower the loss, the longer it will stay off.

- **Believe that you can:** We've all heard the depressing statistic that 98% of people gain back the weight they lose. That alone makes you say, "Why even bother to try?" But, that number is from a 1959 diet study of just 100 obese individuals. More recent studies suggest that the number is much more promising because more than half all people who lose weight lose it on their own. For the past 20 years, the National Weight Control Registry (NWCR) has been tracking more than 10,000 individuals who have lost at least 30 pounds and have kept it off for at least a year (www.nwcr.ws).

- **Stop making excuses:** While it's popular to blame our genes or our metabolism, our weight is mostly determined by our forks and our feet (in other words, how much we eat and how much we move). The more we move, the more muscle mass we have and the higher our metabolic rate. Those "bad genes" may be just plain bad habits that we inherited from our family such as the dislike of vegetables or exercise, our preference for fatty foods and sweets, skipping breakfast, or eating our meals while watching TV. Our bad habits also come from friends, too. The more overweight our friends, the more overweight we are. Realize that fewer than 3% of overweight individuals have a metabolism problem because of their thyroid, and even if that's the cause for the weight gain, the replacement hormone medicine won't make the excess weight melt off. You still have to lose the weight the old fashioned way: by eating less than your body burns. I also hear people blame their excess weight on a problem digesting their food. If this were true, the particles wouldn't be able to pass into the bloodstream, which means that more of it would run through the gastrointestinal tract and into the toilet. If someone were really having a problem digesting food, they would be losing weight, not gaining it.

- **Even small changes matter:** With all the headlines about how heavy we're getting, you'd think we are greatly overeating. But, that isn't true. Think back 10 or 20 years ago (or maybe last year) to recall what you weighed and compare it to what you currently weigh. My guess is that it's fairly close to the average weight gain of about a pound or two a year. Because there are 3500 calories in a pound of fat and 350 days in a year (ha ha, I'm rounding this off for simple math), you can easily see that for every pound we gain a year, it's attributed to overeating just 10 extra calories a day! So, to lose weight, start by making small changes rather than dieting.

- **Move it:** If you've ever looked at the pitifully low number of calories burned on a piece of exercise equipment, you realize that you can't out-exercise a poor diet. But activity is still important. Small movement (such as fidgeting, standing while working, and pacing while on the phone) help to burn a substantial amount of calories over time. And, large movements (like running, biking, and lifting weights) help to build muscle mass, so you'll experience a higher metabolic rate. That means you'll burn more calories 24/7!

- **Focus on protein:** Aim for 20–30 g of protein at every meal (don't forget breakfast) to satiate your appetite. If you're cutting back on calories, keep it closer to 30 g of protein; it will help you keep your muscle mass up.

- **Eat less fat and more fiber:** Sure, cutting back on carbs, proteins, or fats will decrease calories and weight, but can you stick with it? While there's no reason to cut out moderate amounts of fats and alcohol, realize that it's easy to overconsume these calories without them filling you up. Instead, fill up on lower-fat, high-fiber foods such as fruits, vegetables, and whole grains. Popcorn (6 cups has 100 calories) exerts a stronger effect on satiety than 150 calories of potato chips (just 15 chips).

- **Eat on a regular basis:** Skipping or skimping on meals does not lead to weight loss. Remember that breakfast is the most important meal of the day.

- **Be consistent:** We all know people that are "good" during the work week and then "blow it" on the weekends. Others have "on" days when they greatly restrict their calories (or even fast) and "off" days when they can eat whatever they want. Can you lose weight this way? Of course, as long as you cut back on total calories, you'll lose weight on the scale (though not necessarily fat loss). But if you want to ensure long-term maintenance and improved energy, aim for consistency. Among those in the NWCR, people who reported that they ate more consistently across the week (and across the year) were 1.5 times more likely to maintain their weight within five pounds over the subsequent year than those who dieted more strictly on the weekdays.

- **Control portion sizes:** According to Dr. Wansink, portion distortion begins as early as age three, and it affects people of all weights. The more we're served, the more we eat, even when we're not hungry. Dr. Brian Wansink and his team have shown that when restaurants serve large portion sizes, we tend to eat 30–50% more. Large packages encourage us to eat in the range of 20–40% more. That's true even when the food doesn't taste good. Why do larger portion sizes lead us to overeat? It's not just because we have a tendency to clean our plate; portion sizes also create our consumption norms, and we tend to underestimate the calories in large-size portions. Barbara Rolls, another researcher in this field, finds that individuals presented with large portions generally do not report or respond to increased levels of fullness, suggesting that hunger and satiety signals are ignored or overridden.

- **Don't drink your calories:** Chapter 9 discussed the importance of staying hydrated; this is especially important to remember when you're trying to lose weight. So, drink water all day long, especially before and during meals, and you'll eat fewer calories. Studies have shown that when beverages with calories are consumed (alcohol, regular soda, and juice), people tend to eat just as much food, resulting in a greater calorie intake. That's because calorie-laden fluids aren't filling.

- **Slow down:** It may not surprise you to hear that men tend to eat faster than women. One study found that men consumed about 80 calories per minute, while women consumed 52 calories per minute. But did you know that the speed at which we eat may also affect our weight? Several studies demonstrate that slimmer people tend to eat more slowly than heavier people. The faster people ate, the more calories they ate, and the more they tended to weigh. Slower eaters also tend to drink more water at meals, too. So, it makes sense to slow down our eating. Take smaller bites and chew longer before swallowing.

- **Reduce distractions and mindless eating:** As we mentioned in a previous bullet point, the calorie difference related to maintaining weight versus weight gain is miniscule (about 10 calories). Therefore, it's important to stop eating when you're no longer hungry instead of pushing your limit. To better read your hunger level, it helps to reduce distractions that will lead to a general increase in food intake. So, put down that magazine or newspaper and turn off the TV while eating. Groups that practice mindful eating tend to eat fewer calories and lose weight without feeling deprived.

- **Monitor yourself on a regular basis and respond quickly:** Using data from the NWCR participants, researchers found that the weight regained at year one determined how much would be regained at year two. Therefore, once you've lost the weight, it's important to respond quickly to weight gain. That means catching even small weight gains by taking body measurements or weighing yourself on a regular basis to see trends. Others have found success by staying conscious of critical behaviors such as writing down what they eat (this helps even if you're not tracking calories), using a pedometer to count steps, and keeping track of their water intake.

- **Have a plan:** Success is dependent upon having a plan that works for you. Some people decide to limit exposure to high-calorie foods by not buying them. Others use the weekend to plan, shop, and prepare meals and snacks for the coming week.

Appendix E: Breakfast Ideas

Having no time in the morning is no longer a valid excuse for skipping breakfast. Here are some quick and filling breakfast suggestions containing around 300–500 calories, 20–30 g protein, and moderate carbohydrates and fat. Feel free to complete each meal (to match your calorie needs) by eating larger portions or adding fruit or milk.

Peanut Butter on Toasted Whole Wheat English Muffin with Milk

A bagel is loaded with 60 g high GI carbs (the equivalence of 4 slices of bread) and contains about 350 calories. Opt instead to toast one whole grain English muffin and spread each half with 1 tablespoon peanut butter (or other nut butter). Enjoy with glass of nonfat dairy or soymilk to reach 20 g protein. I use freshly ground peanut butter (100% peanuts, no added sugar or salt) from our local grocery store. If not available, opt for natural nut butter without added hydrogenated fats. Just stir and place in refrigerator to prevent the natural healthy oils from separating again.

Scrambled Egg Burrito

Sauté a small amount of chopped onions and peppers (or last night's dinner vegetable) in a skillet. Add two eggs, scramble with a spatula, and cook thoroughly (use ½ cup egg substitute to reduce fat and calories). Place in whole grain flour tortilla (around 120 calories) and sprinkle 1 ounce (or 2 tablespoons) shredded low-fat cheese (I like Cabot's Creamery low-fat cheeses). Two egg whites have as much protein as a whole egg.

Open-Face Tex-Mex Sausage Muffin

Cook two veggie MorningStar Farms Hot & Spicy sausage patties according to package directions. Thinly slice ¼ avocado and layer it over a toasted whole-grain English muffin. Top each half with one sausage patty and 2 tablespoons Newman's Own Black Bean & Corn Salsa (or the salsa of your choice).

Fried Eggs and Beans

Fry two eggs in a skillet with 1 teaspoon canola oil. Serve with ½ cup canned beans (I like Bush's Seasoned Black Beans) and two small corn tortillas (warmed in the microwave).

Bagel and Lox

Top one small toasted whole-grain bagel (or half a large New York-style bagel) with 2 ounces sliced lox, 3 tablespoons low-fat cream cheese, red onion slices, and capers. I like the brand Alternative Bagels.

Higher-Protein Cereal and Milk

Most cereals are low protein and high GI: the opposite of what you need to start your day. To obtain 20 or more grams of protein, select a higher-protein, high-fiber cereal such as Kashi Toasted Berry Crumble Go Lean Crisp (look at the Nutrition Facts panel for a cereal with 6+ protein per serving). Pour a rounded cup of cereal into a bowl and cover with a cup of nonfat milk.

Grab-and-Go Breakfast

Start off with 20 g protein such as 3 hard-cooked eggs, 3 low-fat cheese sticks (such as Sargento Mozzarella sticks), or 1½ ounces of low-fat jerky. Then, add 30–45 g of carbohydrates, like a glass of nonfat milk and a piece of fresh fruit or perhaps a cup of Greek yogurt or a fruit/nut bar such as Lara's Cashew Cookie bar.

Microwaved Breakfast from the Freezer

There are very few frozen breakfast options that contain the minimum of 20 g of protein or more. Amy's Tofu Scramble and Cedarlane Egg White Omelette with Spinach and Mushrooms meets this requirement, but you'll need to add another carb choice (a fruit, a grain like oatmeal, or milk) to bump up the carbs to meet your nutrition needs. The following choices are fairly close to 20 g of protein but tend to be too low in calories to meet one's breakfast needs, so you'll need to add one or more additional carb choices to round out the meal:

- **Good Food Made Simple:** Breakfast Burrito with Eggs, Cheese, & Canadian Bacon

- **Lean Cuisine:** Canadian Bacon or Veggie Egg White on English Muffin Sandwiches

- **Jimmy Dean Delights:** Turkey Sausage, Egg White, Cheese, on English Muffin Sandwich

- **Jimmy Dean Delights:** Canadian Bacon Breakfast Sandwich

- **Morning Star:** Sausage, Egg & Cheese Breakfast Sandwich

- **Special K:** Ham, Egg, and Pepper Jack Cheese Flatbread Sandwich

Oatmeal and Milk To Go

Many restaurants sell oatmeal, but even those with added nuts do not contain adequate protein. To bump it up to close to 20 g protein (but not quite), order a medium-sized steamed nonfat milk with the oatmeal (unprepared). Add about half of the steamed milk to the raw oats, cover, and let sit for 5 minutes. Then, drink the remaining milk (perhaps with a sprinkle of cinnamon). Both McDonald's Fruit and Maple Oatmeal and Starbucks Whole Grain Oatmeal with Fruit and Nuts (no sugar) made this way contain 400–450 calories, contain 16–17 g of protein, and 5–6 g of fiber. And, both are available 24 hours a day.

Dr. Jo's Breakfast in a Cup

If you're a frequent traveler like me, you've found yourself in a place without food options. For example, when you have a 5 a.m. flight and breakfast joints are not yet open, or you arrive at the hotel so late that local restaurants are closed. When traveling, I carry a small insulated cup, a portable immersion heater (purchased from Bed Bath & Beyond for under $10), and several zipper-lock baggies filled with ½ cup quick oats, ½ cup nonfat dried dairy (or soy) milk, a mini box of raisins, 2 tablespoons chopped walnuts, and an optional sweetener. To make my quick breakfast in a cup, fill the insulated cup with 8 ounces water, place the portable immersion heater inside the cup, and plug it in to an electric socket. Once boiling, remove the heater and add the contents of the bag. Let sit for a five minutes and enjoy.

Restaurant Breakfast Sandwich

Each of these suggestions contains 350–490 calories and a minimum of 20 g of protein:

- **Einstein's:** Thintastic Egg White Turkey Sausage Sandwich or Ham & Swiss Egg Sandwich

- **Panera:** Bread Egg White, Avocado, and Spinach Power on Sprouted-Grain Bagel Flat

- **Starbucks:** Ham & Cheddar Breakfast Sandwich
- **Subway:** 6-inch Egg White, Cheese, Ham Sandwich or 6-inch Western Egg and Cheese or 6-inch Sunrise Melt with egg white

Pick Two

Because most other breakfast options do not contain the minimum 20 g of protein, pair it with another option (milk, latte, eggs, or yogurt) to bump up the protein content. Here are some ideas that range from 360–460 calories:

- **Jack in the Box:** Breakfast Jack with carton of 1% lowfat milk
- **McDonald's:** Egg McMuffin with carton of 1% milk
- **McDonald's:** White Delight and small latte
- **McDonald's:** Fruit & Maple Oatmeal with an order of scrambled eggs
- **Starbucks:** Spinach Feta Egg White Breakfast Wrap and small latte
- **Starbucks:** reduced-fat Turkey Bacon Breakfast Sandwich and Greek yogurt with berries parfait

Restaurant Breakfast Options

While many complete breakfast options at restaurants are loaded with 800–1000 calories, the suggestions below contain adequate protein combined with moderate carbs at just 330–560 calories:

- **Denny's:** Fit Slam (scrambled egg white with spinach and grape tomatoes, turkey bacon strips, an English muffin, and seasonal fruit)
- **IHOP:** Simple & Fit Veggie Omelet with fresh fruit
- **IHOP:** Simple & Fit Two-Egg Breakfast
- **IHOP:** Simple & Fit Blueberry Harvest Grain 'N Nut Combo
- **Panera Bread:** Power Breakfast Egg White Bowl with Roasted Turkey and steel-cut oats with blueberries and granola
- **Perkin's:** Spinach and Mushroom Scramble
- **Perkin's:** Banana Whole Wheat French Toast with chicken sausage

Dr. Jo's Homemade Granola

Most granolas are made with a lot of added sugar and fat. This one has just four ingredients. Feel free to customize with different nuts and add dried fruit. Because it's lower in sugar than most of the commercial varieties, it has a crumbly texture, making it perfect for sprinkling on yogurt.

Ingredients

4 cups uncooked quick oats

1 cup raw slivered almonds or chopped walnuts (or a combination)

1/4 cup canola oil

1/3 cup honey

Mix all four ingredients together in a large bowl. Spread the mixture on a baking sheet and bake at 350 degrees for about 10 minutes. Once cooled, stored in a closed container. The recipe makes about 6 cups. Each ½-cup serving of granola contains: 180 calories and 4 g protein. Combine with ½ cup fresh raspberries (or other fruit) and 8 ounces nonfat Greek yogurt (many of the stores sell 32-ounce containers) for a 400-calorie breakfast with long-lasting energy.

Cottage Cheese Pancakes

Regular pancakes, even whole-wheat ones, tend to be high GI because of their low-protein, high-carb ratio. Adding protein powder to the batter makes the pancakes tough. Instead, add cottage cheese for protein. Here's a recipe I've using for decades that tastes so good it doesn't even need syrup.

Ingredients

1 cup whole wheat flour (or half white, half whole wheat)

½ teaspoon baking soda

¼ teaspoon salt (omit if using salted cottage cheese)

2 tablespoons sugar

4 eggs (or 8 egg whites)

1 cup nonfat unsalted cottage cheese

½ cup nonfat milk

2 tablespoons canola oil

Optional: fresh or frozen fruit and nuts

In a large bowl, stir together the dry ingredients. In another bowl, whisk together the remaining wet ingredients (eggs, cottage cheese, milk, and oil). Spray a griddle or skillet with nonstick spray and heat on medium heat. Pour ¼ cup mix for each pancake on to the hot skillet; cook until bubbles form on the surface, then flip the pancake and continue cooking until both sides are lightly browned. Makes about 12 pancakes. Three pancakes contain: 320 calories, 20 g protein, 33 g carbs

Refrigerator Muesli

I first tried muesli in Europe decades ago and loved it. Unfortunately, it was prepared with half-and-half cream, so it was high in fat and low in protein. Here's a much healthier (and just as tasty) alternative. The taste of the Greek yogurt comes through, so pick your favorite flavor and variety. While I frequently add raisins and chopped walnuts (because there's no preparation involved and they're readily available in my cabinet), feel free to experiment with chopped fresh fruit and other nuts.

Ingredients
½ cup raw oats
5.3 ounces Greek yogurt
½ cup nonfat milk
1 tablespoon raisins
1 tablespoon chopped walnuts

In a bowl, combine the raw oats, Greek yogurt, nonfat milk, raisins, and chopped walnuts. Cover and place in the refrigerator overnight. A serving contains: 380 calories, 23g protein, 59g carbs.

Fruit Protein Smoothie

I enjoy a smoothie after a tough workout. While peach and berry blends are my favorite, feel free to substitute fruits to match your taste. Before bananas get overly ripe, I peel them, cut them in half, place them in a freezer bag, and freeze them, so they're always available. I also freeze orange juice in ice cube trays, too (one cube is about 2 tablespoons).

Ingredients
3/4 cup nonfat dairy or soy milk
1/2 cup frozen blueberries (with no added sugar)
1/2 cup frozen peaches (with no added sugar)
2 tablespoons orange juice (with no added sugar)

1/2 banana
3/4 scoop protein powder (my favorite is Jay Robb vanilla-
    flavored egg protein)
Combine all ingredients in a blender and blend until smooth.
One smoothie contains: 300 calories, 24g protein, 50g carbs.

Beef Sticky Buns

A twist on cinnamon buns, these savory buns get a protein boost from homemade beef breakfast sausage and plenty of veggies like mushrooms and spinach. Yet, two Beef Sticky Buns contain just 410 calories, 28 g protein, 53 g carbs, and 10 g fat. Recipe courtesy of The Beef Checkoff (www.BeefItsWhatsForDinner.com).

Ingredients
1 recipe basic country beef breakfast sausage (recipe below)
1 cup sliced button mushrooms
3/4 cup diced onion
3 cups fresh baby spinach
1/2 cup reduced-fat shredded cheddar cheese
1 package (13.8 ounces) refrigerated pizza dough (whole
    wheat, if available.

- Prepare the basic country beef breakfast sausage. Set aside 2 cups of beef in a large bowl; reserve the remaining beef for another use.

- Add onion and mushrooms to the same skillet and cook over medium heat, 5–7 minutes or until the vegetables are tender, stirring occasionally. Add the spinach to the skillet and stir to wilt the spinach. Add the vegetable mixture to the beef and set aside 20–25 minutes or until mixture is cooled completely, stirring occasionally. Stir in cheese.

- Preheat oven to 425° F. Unroll the pizza dough on a flat surface. Pat or roll the dough evenly into a 14x10-inch rectangle, pinching together any tears, if necessary. Spread the beef mixture onto dough, leaving a ½-inch border on the short side furthest from you. Starting at the closest short end, roll up jelly-roll style, pinching the dough to close. Slice the dough into 8 pieces using a serrated knife and careful sawing motion; place cut side up on greased baking sheet.

- Bake at 425° F for 18–20 minutes or until golden brown. Remove buns to cooling rack.

Basic Country Beef Breakfast Sausage
Ingredients
1 pound ground beef (96% lean)
2 teaspoons chopped fresh sage or ½ teaspoon rubbed sage
1 teaspoon garlic powder
1 teaspoon onion powder
½ teaspoon salt
¼ to ½ teaspoon crushed red pepper

Combine all ingredients in a large bowl, mixing lightly but thoroughly. Heat a large nonstick skillet over medium-high heat. Add beef mixture and cook 8–10 minutes, breaking into ½-inch crumbles and stirring occasionally. (Cooking times are for fresh or thoroughly thawed ground beef. Ground beef should be cooked to an internal temperature of 160° F. Color is not a reliable indicator of doneness.) Makes 2½ cups crumbles.

Appendix F: Lunch Ideas

Sandwich from Home

The most common lunchtime meal is a sandwich with just a few thin slices of meat, a soda, plus chips or cookies (or both). Unfortunately, this results in a low-protein, high-GI meal unlikely to effectively fuel you through the afternoon. To REBOOT your sandwich, choose whole wheat bread (make sure the first ingredient is a whole grain) and add at least 2 ounces of quality deli meat and/ or low-fat cheese to boost the protein to about 20 g. Note: this is a lot more meat than most of us add to a sandwich; a pound of meat would make just eight sandwiches.

There are many low-fat deli meat choices including turkey, turkey pastrami, chicken, ham, and roast beef. For added nutrition (and a satisfying crunch factor) top the sandwich with plenty of veggies including lettuce, tomato, and onion. Dress your sandwich with a thin smear of mustard or mayo plus a piece of fresh fruit or salad. Because bread (even whole-grain bread) is still a fairly high-GI option, you may want to cut the sandwich in half and add a cup of protein-rich bean edamame or soup (such as split pea, black bean, or lentil), milk, yogurt, or some hummus to dip raw veggies into to ensure a lower-GI meal (and subsequently, minimize the mid-afternoon slump).

Grab a Sub to Go

Many small (6-inch) subs can fit into the REBOOT specs for carbs. Though, to get enough protein, you might need to double up on the meat, select an item with larger meat portions, or add cheese. Even if you need more calories, it's best not to order a larger sub because it will contain too many carbs (especially because bread is high GI). Instead, add a carton of milk and a piece of fruit. When ordered without optional ingredients such as cheese, mayo, oil, and dressing, the sandwiches below contain 310–440 calories, 20–29 g of protein, and 23–66 g of carbs. Count on anywhere from 50–100 calories extra for each of those optional ingredients.

- **Firehouse Sub:** Hook & Ladder Lite or Turkey Salsa Verde

- **Jason's Deli's:** Deli Club (half) or Mediterranean Wrap

- **Jimmy John's:** #2 Big John (roast beef) or #4 Turkey Tom on 7-Grain Bread

- **Quizno's:** Honey Bourbon Chicken Flatbread, Honey Bourbon Chicken Small Sub, or Quizno's Turkey Lite Small Sub

- **Subway:** 6-inch Club Sandwich, Oven-Roasted Chicken, or Sweet Onion Teriyaki Sandwich

- **Wawa:** Double Meat Turkey, Ham, or Roast Beef on Whole Wheat Short Roll

Pick Two

Sometimes a whole sandwich has too many high-GI carbs, so it's better to order half a sandwich plus another option. Try these combos at 380–545 calories, 23–32 g of protein, 49–68 g of carbs, and 10–23 g of fat:

- **Jason's Deli:** Amy's Turkey-O Sandwich (half) plus three-bean salad

- **Panera Bread:** Pick Two: half Smoked Ham & Swiss Sandwich plus a cup of Vegetable Pesto Soup or half Tuna Salad Sandwich on Honey Wheat plus a cup of Black Bean Soup or Thai Chicken Flatbread plus Thai Chicken Salad with Thai vinaigrette

- **Wendy's:** half-size Apple Pecan Chicken Salad plus a small chili (no crackers or cheese)

Salad

A salad from home is a good choice for lunch, as long as it contains the minimum 20 g of protein and adequate calories. Unfortunately, too many people pack only vegetables with fat-free dressing, which doesn't provide nearly enough calories to last the next few hours. Here's the key: start with a good variety of vegetables, plus 20 g of protein in the form of meat, poultry, fish, eggs, and cheese. Then, add the appropriate amount of carbs for you such as fruit, beans, whole grain crackers. Because fat doesn't satiate us, it's important to keep your dressing choice to about 100 calories. That's about two tablespoons of vinaigrette or twice as much of a low-fat dressing.

A salad-only meal from a restaurant is usually of two extremes. When the calories are moderate, it's usually too low in protein and calories. On the other hand, many restaurant salads are over 1000 calories once you add in the dressings. Here are some that are both moderate in calories (325–515 calories) yet higher in protein (21–37 g) and moderate in carbs (30–66 g):

- **Applebee's:** Thai Shrimp Salad
- **Chipotle:** Lettuce Salad (no shell) with barbacoa, choice of beans, brown rice, and salsa
- **Jack in the Box:** Grilled Chicken Salad with low-fat balsamic dressing and croutons
- **Qdoba Mexican Grill:** Naked Salad (no tortilla) with grilled chicken, cilantro-lime dressing, pico de gallo, black beans, and fajita vegetables
- **Steak 'n Shake:** Apple Pecan Salad with grilled chicken and reduced-fat balsamic vinaigrette

Frozen Dinners

When you examine the nutrition information, you'll notice that most frozen dinners marketed as healthful are too low in protein; many have only 10 g or less. And, most are too low in calories to be filling. Let's face it: 200 calories isn't going to fill you up for very long. Here are a few options that have around 300 calories (290–440), 20–27 g of protein, and moderate fat (7–15 g) and carbs (28–69 g):

- **Lean Cuisine:** Pomegranate Chicken, Chicken Club Panini, or Dinnertime Collection Salisbury Steak with Potatoes and Carrots
- **Lyfe Kitchen:** Orange Mango Chicken or Chicken Chile Verde with Polenta and Black Beans
- **Michael Angelo's:** Spaghetti with Meatballs or Chicken Parmesan
- **Saffron Road:** Lemongrass Basil Chicken or Chicken Pad Thai with Rice Noodles
- **Tandoor Chef:** Chicken Curry with Seasoned Basmati Rice
- **Weight Watchers:** Chicken Fettuccine

One of my favorite frozen dinners is Amy's Tortilla Casserole & Black Beans Bowl. It contains 390 calories (that's good), but just 17 g protein, so I bump up the protein by adding a glass of milk, a latte, or a cup of yogurt.

Shelf-Stable Meals

Want a shelf-stable well-balanced meal to keep in your desk? Most shelf-stable meals don't contain enough protein. Here's my favorite combination of two items that does – light tuna plus a cup of bean soup. If I'm concerned about a tight plane connection, or if I have back-to-back meetings and presentations (with no time for meals), I throw these into my suitcase. While there are plenty of shelf-stable tuna and chicken pouches or cans, most of the salad options are too low in protein, and other options including just tuna or chicken require you to purchase other items to make them a complete meal (making packing more complicated). These tuna options contain 200–230 calories, 18–20 g of protein, 17–20 g of carbs, and 7–9 g of fat:

- **Starkist:** Charlie's Lunch Kit (light tuna in a can, crackers, reduced-calorie mayonnaise, and relish)

- **Starkist:** Lunch To Go (light tuna in a pouch, reduced-calorie mayonnaise, relish, and a spoon)

- **Bumble Bee:** Sensations Seasoned Tuna Medley with crackers (three flavors: Sundried Tomato & Basil, Lemon & Pepper, or Spicy Thai Chili)

For a high-protein bean soup that doesn't require a can opener and a microwave, opt for Nile Spice or McDougall soups available in paper cups (similar to the ramen noodle products). Choose the lentil, black bean, or split pea soups. I usually pack an insulated cup and portable immersion heater to heat the water. Those paper cups are too bulky to pack, so I portion one serving of the soup into plastic baggies (check the label as most cups contain two servings). One serving of these soups contains 120–170 calories, 8–10 g of protein, 21–35 g of carbs, and 1 g of fat:

- **Dr. McDougall's:** Black Bean & Lime or Vegan Split Pea Soup

- **Nile Spice:** Red Beans and Rice or Lentil Soup

Grilled Chicken Sandwich

Most grilled chicken sandwiches from fast food restaurants provide a good blend of adequate calories, proteins, and carbs. These contain 320–460 calories, 23–34 g of protein, 32–50 g of carbs, and 5–17 g of fat (the higher fat ones have mayonnaise or sauces, which you can cut out):

- **Burger King:** Tendergrill Chicken Sandwich without mayonnaise

- **Carl's Jr.:** Charbroiled BBQ Chicken Sandwich

- **Chick-Fil-A:** Grilled Chicken Sandwich

- **Einstein's:** Thintastic Chicken Pesto Sandwich

- **Hardee's:** Charbroiled BBQ Chicken Sandwich

- **McDonald's:** Grilled Chicken Classic Sandwich

- **Sonic:** Grilled Chicken Sandwich

- **Wendy's:** Ultimate Chicken Grill Sandwich

- **WhatABurger:** Grilled Chicken Sandwich

Other Restaurant Sandwiches, Wraps, Tacos, and More

Here are some additional lunch choices with 320–540 calories, 21–42 g of protein, 30–71 g of carbs, and 8–18 g of fat:

- **Arby's:** Roast Beef Classic

- **Burger King:** BK Veggie without mayonnaise

- **Chick-Fil-A:** Grilled Chicken Cool Wraps without dressing

- **Chipotle:** three soft corn tortillas with chicken or steak, choice of beans, and salsa

- **Einstein's:** Honey-Glazed Smoked Salmon Sandwich

- **Hardee's:** Original Turkey Burger

- **Jack in the Box:** Chicken Fajita Pita with salsa

- **Panda Express:** Grilled Asian or Teriyaki Chicken entrée with mixed vegetables as the side (instead of rice)

- **Perkin's:** Roast Turkey Sandwich

- **Qdoba Mexican Grill:** three crispy tacos with shredded beef, salsa, and lettuce

- **Qdoba Mexican Grill:** three soft flour-tortilla tacos with grilled steak, pico de gallo, lettuce, and fajita vegetables

- **Starbucks:** Chicken Santa Fe Panini or Ham & Swiss Panini

- **Taco Bell:** two Fresco chicken or grilled steak soft tacos

Pizza

Pizza can be tricky. For most varieties, in order to get at least 20 g of protein, you'd need to order three slices of pizza, but then you'd be getting too many calories and carbs. Here are some options that fit the protein/carb REBOOT specs (380–580 calories, 20–26 g protein, and 46–66 g carbs):

- **Papa John's:** medium original-crust Hawaiian BBQ Chicken (two slices)

- **Papa John's:** large thin-crust Hawaiian BBQ Chicken (two slices)

- **Pizza Hut:** large thin-crust Veggie Lover's Pizza (two slices)

- **Pizza Hut:** medium thin-crust Chicken Supreme Pizza (two slices)

Half Now, Half Later

You'll notice that many of the other restaurant lunch choices listed above are from fast food joints because most of the lunch offerings from casual restaurants contain 1000 calories or more! Unless you're running marathons, that calorie load is likely to cause a mid-afternoon energy slump. When dining out at these restaurants, opt to split a meal with a friend, or eat half of the dish for lunch and save the other half for another lunch (or for your afternoon goûter). Below are some of the lower-calorie options, but still a half portion contains 480–615 calories, 24–30 g of protein, 55–80 g of carbs, and 10–25 g of fat:

- **Applebee's:** Roast Beef, Bacon and Mushroom Melt (half portion) plus a side of seasonal vegetables

- **California Pizza Kitchen:** Original BBQ Chicken Pizza and Asparagus and Arugula Salad (half portions for everything)

- **Chili's:** Grilled Chicken Sandwich with fries (half of everything)

- **TGI Friday's:** Jack Daniel's Chicken Sandwich (half the sandwich, no side)

Appendix G: Dinner Ideas

The easiest way to plan your REBOOT dinner meal is in three simple steps. First, choose your protein (beef, chicken, fish, shellfish, or veggie protein) in a portion containing 20–30 g of protein. A piece of meat about the size of a deck of cards contains 21 g of protein; if you're choosing a nonmeat protein (such as tofu or beans), check the label for the appropriate portion size. Next, add one (or, even better, a variety of) carbs using the portion sizes listed in Chapter 8. Recall that a 400-calorie meal includes about 45 g of carbs. Lastly, add some veggies. Here are several 400-calorie dinner options:

Protein	Carbs (around 45 g)	Veggies
Grilled chicken	Piece fresh fruit 1 cup butternut squash	1 cup green beans
Sirloin steak	½ cup potatoes Whole grain roll 1 cup milk	1 cup steamed broccoli
Lean ground beef	1 cup pasta ½ cup spaghetti sauce	Small green salad
Salmon	1 cup brown rice	1 cup green/yellow
squash		
Tofurkey	1 flour tortilla 1 cup black beans	1 cup carrots

Chipotle Three-Bean Veggie Chili

Some meals have all three key components (protein, carbs, and veggies) in one pot. This vegetarian chili developed by Allison Stevens, personal chef and registered dietitian nutritionist (RDN), is simple to make and requires only 10 minutes prep time, plus 30–60 minutes to cook. Feel free to use lower-sodium beans to reduce the sodium content. One recipe makes four hearty servings, each containing 350 calories, 20 g of protein, 58 g of carbs, and 9 g of fat. Allison's company, PrepDish.com, offers recipes, meal plans with shopping lists, and detailed instructions for prep day, so you can serve delicious meals during the week in no time flat. While she focuses on gluten-free options, I like it because it broadens my ideas beyond my usual meal choices.

Ingredients

1 dried chipotle pepper
1 teaspoon canola oil
1 green bell pepper
1 yellow bell pepper
1 red bell pepper
½ onion
1 tablespoon chopped garlic
28-ounce can fire-roasted tomatoes
15-ounce can black beans
15-ounce can pinto beans
15-ounce can kidney beans
2–3 tablespoons chili powder
Salt and pepper, to taste
½ cup shredded low-fat cheddar cheese

- Place dried chipotle pepper in 3 cups of hot water and allow to rehydrate. Finely dice the three bell peppers.

- In a large stock pan, sauté the onion, garlic, and three bell peppers in the canola oil.

- Remove and discard the seeds and stem from the rehydrated chipotle pepper (optional: use a few seeds if desired for added heat). Place the chipotle pepper in a blender with 2 cups of hot water and blend until smooth, adding seeds as desired (do so gradually and taste for heat before adding to chili). Add the pureed chili mixture to sautéed veggies.

- Add the fire-roasted tomatoes, 2 tablespoons chili powder, and three cans of beans. Bring to a boil, and then lower the heat to medium-low, stirring occasionally and adding water or chicken or vegetable stock as needed. Continue to cook for 30 minutes to 1 hour. Season to taste with chili powder, salt, and pepper. Serve hot and sprinkle 2 tablespoons of shredded cheese on each bowl.

Dinner Meals Out

With most restaurant entrees at 1000 calories or more (that's before drinks, appetizers, bread, or dessert), it's easy to pack on the pounds and create an energy slump when dining out. Here are some sensible options to try instead:

- **Applebee's:** While options are constantly changing, check out the Weight Watchers and Have it All Options section of the menu.
  - Weight Watchers Lemon Parmesan Shrimp (510 calories, 30 g protein, 65 g carbs, 15 g fat)
  - Napa Chicken & Portobellos (480 calories, 54 g protein, 35 g carbs, 14 g fat)
- **Boston Market:** When you start with chicken or turkey, there are plenty of mix-and-match options to meet your needs. Remove the chicken skin for added calorie and fat savings.
  - Quarter White Rotisserie Chicken without skin, green beans, garlic dill new potatoes, cornbread without butter (570 calories, 55 g protein, 60 g carbs, 14 g fat)
- **California Pizza Kitchen:** Sometimes an appetizer is plenty of food.
  - Shrimp Lettuce Wraps (480 calories, 25 g protein, 40 g carbs, 23 g fat)
- **Cheesecake Factory:** Stick with the SKINNYLISCIOUS menu for options at 590 calories or less, such as:
  - White Chicken Chili (580 calories, 56 g protein, 41 g carbs, 19 g fat)
  - Chicken & Mushroom Lettuce Wraps (350 calories, 23 g protein, 27 g carbs, 16 g fat)
  - Edamame (to add as a side or enjoy as a snack, it contains 290 calories, 24 g protein, 27 g carbs, 9 g fat)
- **Chili's:** Look for the Lighter Choice menu items including:
  - Salmon with sides (540 calories, 47 g protein, 38 g carbs, 24 g fat)
  - Mango-Chile Tilapia with sides (560 calories, 38 g protein, 57 g carbs, 21 g fat)
  - Margarita Grilled Chicken with sides (610 calories, 51 g protein, 67 g carbs, 16 g fat)

- **Olive Garden:** Look for the Lighter Fare sections of the menu, which are constantly changing. Here are some current Lighter Fare entrée options (not including breadstick, soup, or salad):

  - Seafood Brodetto (480 calories, 47 g protein, 35 g carbs, 16 g fat)

  - Garden Capellini Pomodoro with chicken (570 calories, 38 g protein, 69 g carbs, 14 g fat)

  - Garlic Rosemary Chicken (400 calories, 36 g protein, 29 g carbs, 16 g fat)

- **On the Border Mexican Grill:** Look for Border Smart menu options such as:

  - Grilled Chicken Fajitas (550 calories, 50 g protein, 65 g carbs, 10 g fat)

  - Grilled Chicken Fajita Tacos with a side order of black beans (480 calories, 34 g protein, 64 g carbs, 10 g fat)

  - Mango Chicken Salad with fat-free mango-citrus vinaigrette (400 calories, 34 g protein, 52 g carbs, 6 g fat)

- **Outback Steakhouse:** The menu has plenty of nutritionally balanced options including:

  - Victoria's 6-ounce filet, sweet potatoes, and fresh steamed green beans (540 calories, 41 g protein, 63 g carbs, 15 g fat)

  - Grilled Shrimp on the Barbie (appetizer portion) with rice and broccoli (sides) (680 calories, 36 g protein, 65 g carbs, 28 g fat)

  - Simply Mahi and Green Beans (435 calories, 53 g protein, 39 g carbs, 7 g fat)

- **PF Chang's:** Because of their high-caloric content, most of the menu items are best shared. In addition, dishes can often be made lower in fat and calories by requesting they be prepared "stock-velveted," which means using stock instead of oil to stir-fry. Here are a few options that fit into the REBOOT guidelines:

  - Chicken Lettuce Wraps (530 calories, 32 g protein, 47 g carbs, 24 g fat)

  - Steamed Budda's Feast with a half order of brown rice (415 calories, 29 g protein, 65 g carbs, 5 g fat)

  - Ginger Chicken with Broccoli with a half order of brown rice (625 calories, 62 g protein, 71 g carbs, 12 g fat)

- **Red Lobster:** For sensibility, there's a Lighthouse menu, and fish is available in half portions as well.
  - Wood-Grilled Lobster, Shrimp, and Scallops with rice and broccoli (390 calories, 43 g protein, 41 g carbs, 6 g fat)
  - Lighthouse Wood-Grilled Rainbow Trout with rice and asparagus (420 calories, 34 g protein, 44 g carbs, 15 g fat)
  - Steamed Maine Lobster with corn, potatoes, and a salad with red wine vinaigrette (670 calories, 64 g protein, 61 g carbs, 20 g fat)
- **Ruby Tuesday:** Look for the Fit & Trim and Petite Plate options including:
  - Hickory Bourbon Salmon with grilled zucchini and roasted spaghetti squash (485 calories, 44 g protein, 25 g carbs, 23 g fat)
  - Hickory Bourbon Chicken with grilled zucchini and roasted spaghetti squash (450 calories, 43 g protein, 25 g carbs, 10 g fat)
- **TGIFriday's:** Most items are so high calorie that they are best split. Here's one entree that's reasonably sized:
  - Sizzling Chicken and Spinach or Sizzling Sirloin and Spinach (the full order averages 410 calories, 50 g protein, 15 g carbs, 17 g fat)

Appendix H: Snack Ideas

CARB SNACKS

Carbs are digested and absorbed in two hours or less, so they won't provide enough fuel for a large gap between meals. But, they are enough to tide you over for an hour or two, until your next meal, or before a workout. Some people also eat fruit on long activities such as hikes or bike rides as a healthier option to sugar-rich fluid-replacement beverages. Of course, be sure to drink with plenty of water.

Fruit

Fresh fruit, dried fruit, or canned fruit contain no protein but have about 100 calories and 15–20 g of carbs. Here are some approximate 100-calorie portions:

- Small banana
- Medium-sized apple, peach, or pear
- Large orange
- ½ grapefruit
- ¾ cup fruit juice
- 1 cup black- or blueberries
- 1 cup canned fruit (packed in water or its own syrup)
- 1½ cup grapes, melons, or strawberries
- 2 clementines or plums
- 5 small apricots
- 3 tablespoons dried fruit (a small box of raisins, 4 prunes, 2 peach halves, 4 apple rings)

Popcorn

Chips tend to be high in fat and low in fiber. Popcorn is a much healthier option with more fiber and low-GI carbs. I make mine the old fashioned way: with a thin layer of canola oil in a heavy pan. There are microwavable options of all sizes to fit your calorie needs. Watch out for movie theater popcorn; most theaters cook theirs in coconut oil, which contains nearly all saturated fat. A small-size bag contains about 450 calories and 32 g of fat (24 g of saturated fat), which is as much fat as about a third of a stick of butter.

PROTEIN SNACKS

When your energy is dropping and your hunger level is down to zero, realize that your body is already in the process of increasing your blood glucose from body stores (including muscle protein). Instead of adding to the glucose load, grab some protein to help stabilize your glucose levels. Each of the suggestions below contains around 70–100 calories, at least 7 g of protein, and little or no carbs (check the Nutrition Facts label for more information):

- 1 ounce jerky (beef, turkey, and even ostrich meats are available)
- 1–2 ounces of leftover beef, chicken, fish, etc. (perhaps wrapped in a lettuce leaf)
- 1 ounce low-fat cheese (check out cheese sticks)
- Hard-cooked egg
- ½ cup low-fat cottage cheese
- Individually sized pouch or can of tuna
- Half of an Epic Bar (made with beef, bison, turkey, or lamb and fruits)
- Veggie patty (there's a wide variety made by MorningStar Farms)
- A scoop of protein powder mixed in water (I like the taste of Jay Robb egg white protein)

BALANCED SNACKS

The following snacks provide long-lasting energy with a good balance of carbs to fuel your brain and protein to keep your blood sugar stable.

Milk

Milk (preferably nonfat dairy or soy) is a well-balanced snack; one cup contains about 8 g protein, 12 g carbs, and 80 calories. If you're on the road, there are many places to pick up a small 8-ounce carton including fast food and convenience stores. Keep in mind that almond, hemp, and coconut milk are not good REBOOT snacks because they contain insignificant amounts of protein; most of the calories come from sugar. If you like almond milk, some stores now offer a fortified almond milk containing 5–6 g protein.

Latte

At a coffee shop? A small latte prepared with nonfat milk or soymilk contains about the same nutritional value as one cup of milk mentioned above and approximately 100 calories. Of course, adding sugar and syrup will substantially increase the sugar content and calories; choose sugar-free syrup and use noncaloric sweeteners instead.

Yogurt

Check the label for specifics because yogurts range from low-sugar, lower-calorie products to very-high-calorie ones. For lasting energy, try Greek yogurt. It contains twice as much protein as regular yogurt, and there are many options at 100–150 calories including Chobani, Dannon, Yoplait, and Oikos. While the regular yogurts have 4–7 g protein, the Greek varieties range from 10–13 g for the smaller cups. On-the-road options include:

- **McDonald's:** Fruit 'n Yogurt Parfait with granola (150 calories, 4 g protein, and 30 g carbs.)

- **McDonald's:** Snack Size Fruit & Walnut Salad (210 calories, 4 g protein, 31g carbs)

- **Starbucks:** Greek Yogurt with Berries Parfait (220 calories, 14 g protein, 6 g carbs)

Oatmeal

Most instant oatmeal packages are low in protein and high in sugar. Try Dr. Jo's Breakfast in a Cup (Appendix E) or check out Quaker Weight Control instant oatmeal. Prepared with water it contains 160 calories and 7 g protein, but if you make it with milk, there's 15 g protein and 220 calories. If you're on the road and looking for a more filling snack, many restaurants offer oatmeal (Starbucks and McDonalds offer it 24 hours a day). Even when you skip the sugar, a portion is likely to be in the 250-calorie range with about 6 g protein. You can boost the protein content by asking them to prepare it using steamed milk.

Cup of Soup

While many soups are loaded with sodium, there are a lot of new lower-sodium varieties hitting the stores. Look for soups that contain around 100–150 calories per cup (too low and you won't get enough fuel) and with at least 6 g of protein. One cup of Camp-bell's Chunky Split Pea and Progresso Lentil Soup, for example, contains about 150 calories and 8–12 g of protein. On the road you'll find plenty of smaller-sized soup options with 80–180 calo-ries and 6–13 g of protein including Panera Chicken Noodle and Vegetarian Black Bean Soup, Chick-Fil-A small Chicken Noodle Soup, or Wendy's small Chili. This nutrition information does not include optional items such as bread, crackers, and cheese.

Nuts and Seeds

While we often think of nuts and seeds as being high in pro-tein, more than half of the calories come from fat, even for the dry-roasted varieties. Because fat is so dense in calories, that means that just one handful can easily add up to 200 calories or more. You might want to pull out the measuring cup to portion out nuts into individual baggies: ¼ cup contains 130–205 calories. On the low end are soy nuts (130 calories, 10 g protein). The rest contain 2–7 g protein and 160 calories or more. This includes almonds, cashews, hazelnuts, macadamia nuts, peanuts, pecans, pistachio nuts, and walnuts, as well as sunflower and pumpkin seeds.

For variety, try Emerald Cinnamon- or Cocoa-Roasted Al-monds. Like chocolate? For about 150 calories, you can have 12 Peanut M&Ms, 8 chocolate-covered almonds, 6 Hershey's Kisses with almonds, or 3 miniature Reese's Peanut Butter Cups.

Trail Mix

Nuts and dried fruit can be combined for a great-tasting snack. Use your quarter-cup measuring container and measure out half nuts and half dried fruit. Try raisins and peanuts, cashews and dried cherries, or almonds and apricots. Planters brand sells a variety of prepared fruit-and-nut mixes in individual bags containing about 250 calories per bag. I've found Planters Trail Mix, Planters NU-Trition Apple Cinnamon, and more.

Smoothie

While fruit is healthy, once it's liquefied with sugar added (like most smoothies), you end up with a quickly absorbed, high-GI, high-calorie product. These 300-calorie smoothies would be a more balanced option after an intense workout:

- **Jamba Juice:** Some small-sized drinks contain around 300 calories and 10–16 g protein and around 55–65 g carbs (including Carrot-Orange or Kale-Ribbean Whole Food Nutrition Smoothies, Fit'N Fruitful Smoothies, or Protein Berry Workout)

- **Starbucks:** Chocolate Smoothie contains: 300 calories, 20 g protein, and 53 g carbs

Bars

In the grocery store, you'll find snack and meal bars ranging from 100 calories to several hundreds of calories. I'm always on the lookout for those that contain at least 4 g protein and aren't loaded with sugar. For this reason, I avoid the traditional granola or so-called fruit bars. My favorites are Lara bars because most of them are made with just fruit and nuts. If I feel like I need more protein, I opt for Balance, Kashi, Nature Valley Protein, and Zing bars. For something more savory (rather than sweet), try Epic bars made of meat (bison, beef, turkey, or lamb) and fruit. If you have specific nutrition or food-allergy needs, check out YouBar.com, where you can custom build your bars. While not every product is listed, here's a brief rundown to help you decide which ones to buy. You'll find you love the taste of some and hate others. And, while some make you feel satisfied, others may not.

- **100–120 calories:** If you don't need many calories for your snack and it's difficult to stop at just a half of a bar, look for Lara, Clif KidZ, or Kind Snacks in their mini-size portion. Sam's and Costco stores typically offer these.

- **130–170 calories:** While it depends on the flavor, Clif Builder Snack Bar, Detour, InBar, Kashi, Quaker Medleys, Soy Joy, and True bars tend to be in this calorie range. Protein varies from just 3 g up to 15 g (Detour and InBar are on the higher end).

- **180–250 calories:** The higher-calorie bars include Balance, Cave Man, Clif, Epic, Evolution Harvest, Kind, Kit's, Lara, Luna, Nature Valley Protein, Oh Yeah, PowerCrunch Original Protein Energy, Square Bar, and Zing.

Creative Combos

There are so many ways to make a protein/carb combination snack. Here are some ideas containing around 150 calories:

- ½ cup cottage cheese and a small fresh peach
- ¼ cup hummus and ½ cup raw broccoli
- Low-fat cheese stick and a small pear
- 80–100-calorie yogurt and ½ cup fresh berries
- ¾ cup All Bran wheat flakes and ¾ cup nonfat milk
- ½ English muffin, toasted, with 1 tablespoon peanut butter
- 1 tablespoon almond butter on apple slices
- Ants on a stick: A celery stalk topped with 1 tablespoon peanut butter and 2 tablespoons raisins
- ½ peanut butter sandwich using 1 slice whole wheat bread and 1 tablespoon peanut butter
- 1 ounce Beanitos (about 12 chips) with salsa; these chips are made from beans and contain 4 g protein (my favorite are the Black Bean Beanitos)

These options are in the range of 200–250 calories:

- Yogurt and granola: Sprinkle 2 tablespoons of Dr. Jo's Granola (Appendix E) in a 100–120-calorie cup of yogurt
- ¾ cup Kashi Go Lean Crisp cereal with ¾ cup nonfat milk
- ½ peanut butter and jelly sandwich with 1 slice whole wheat bread, 1 tablespoon peanut butter, and ½ tablespoon jam or jelly
- Milk and cookies: If you take a fiber supplement, try 2 Metamucil wafers (containing psyllium husks) with a cup of nonfat milk
- Charlie's Light Lunch consisting of a can of light tuna, 6 crackers, relish, and light mayonnaise

Snacks on the Go

If you're on the road, check out these many options. These fast-food options contain about 150 calories and 10–12 g protein:

- **Del Taco:** chicken or steak Taco del Carbon

- **Dunkin' Donuts:** Egg White Veggie or Turkey Wake-Up Wrap

- **Taco Bell:** Fresco-Style Grilled Steak or Chicken Soft Taco

- **Taco Bell:** Black Beans & Rice (180 calories, 6 g protein)

Small fast-food sandwiches contain 210–250 calories and 10–15 g protein

- **Arby's Jr:** Roast Beef Sandwich

- **Burger King:** Whopper Jr (no mayonnaise)

- **McDonald's:** hamburger

- **Wendy's Jr.:** hamburger, or Wawa Turkey, Ham, or Roast Beef on a Junior Whole Wheat Roll

These fast-food options contain around 250-280 calories and 16-19 g protein:

- **Dunkin' Donuts:** Egg White Veggie or Turkey Sausage Flatbread

- **McDonald's:** Grilled Chicken Chipotle or Honey Mustard Snack Wraps

- **McDonald's:** Egg White Delite

- **Wendy's:** Grilled Chicken Go Wrap

- **Starbucks:** Chicken & Hummus Bistro Box contains 270 calories and 20 g protein

Protein-Powered Snack Bites

This recipe, courtesy of Daisy Brand Cottage Cheese, combines a few simple ingredients.

Ingredients

4 regular or 12 mini brown-rice cakes

4 tablespoons salt-free almond butter

¾ cup Daisy Brand cottage cheese

1 cup fresh seasonal fruit, thinly sliced

Pinch cinnamon

Spread each rice cake with almond butter and cottage cheese, dividing evenly. Cover with slices of seasonal fruit and a dusting of cinnamon. Serves 4 (1 regular or 3 mini rice cakes). Each serving contains: 190 calories, 9 g protein, 17 g carbs, 11 g fat

References

While more than 1300 articles were reviewed in the research process, the references in the list below were the most helpful in writing REBOOT:

Chapter 1: The Reboot Solution

Dawson D, Reid K. Fatigue, alcohol and performance impairment. Nature. 1997 Jul 17;388(6639):235

Goetzel RZ, Long SR, Ozminkowski RJ, Hawkins K, Wang S, Lynch W. Health, absence, disability, and presenteeism cost estimates of certain physical and mental health conditions affecting U.S. employers. J Occup Environ Med. 2004 Apr;46(4):398-412

Hemp P. Presenteeism: at work--but out of it. Harv Bus Rev. 2004 Oct;82(10):49-58, 155

Institute of Medicine. To Err is Human: Building a Safer Health System. 1999

Janssen N, Kant IJ, Swaen GM, Janssen PP, Schröer CA. Fatigue as a predictor of sickness absence: results from the Maastricht cohort study on fatigue at work. Occup Environ Med. 2003 Jun;60 Suppl 1:i71-6

Johns G. Presenteeism in the workplace: A review and research agenda. J Organiz Behav 2009;31:519-542

Loeppke R, Taitel M, Haufle V, Parry T, Kessler RC, Jinnett K. Health and productivity as a business strategy: a multiemployer study. J Occup Environ Med. 2009 Apr;51(4):411-28

Loeppke R, Taitel M, Richling D, Parry T, Kessler RC, Hymel P, Konicki D. Health and productivity as a business strategy. J Occup Environ Med. 2007 Jul;49(7):712-21

Ricci JA, Chee E, Lorandeau AL, Berger J. Fatigue in the U.S. workforce: prevalence and implications for lost productive work time. J Occup Environ Med. 2007 Jan;49(1):1-10.

Rosenthal TC, Majeroni BA, Pretorius R, Malik K. Fatigue: an overview. Am Fam Physician. 2008 Nov 15;78(10):1173-9. Review

Williamson AM, Feyer AM. Moderate sleep deprivation produces impairments in cognitive and motor performance equivalent to legally prescribed levels of alcohol intoxication. Occup Environ Med. 2000 Oct;57(10):649-55

Chapter 2: All About Sleep

Aldabal L, Bahammam AS. Metabolic, endocrine, and immune consequences of sleep deprivation. Open Respir Med J. 2011;5:31-43

Baron KG, Reid KJ, Kern AS, Zee PC. Role of sleep timing in caloric intake and BMI. Obesity (Silver Spring). 2011 Jul;19(7):1374-81

Benedict C, Brooks SJ, O'Daly OG, Almèn MS, Morell A, Åberg K, Gingnell M, Schultes B, Hallschmid M, Broman JE, Larsson EM, Schiöth HB. Acute sleep deprivation enhances the brain's response to hedonic food stimuli: an fMRI study. J Clin Endocrinol Metab. 2012 Mar;97(3):E443-7

Cizza G, Requena M, Galli G, de Jonge L. Chronic sleep deprivation and seasonality: implications for the obesity epidemic. J Endocrinol Invest. 2011 Nov;34(10):793-800

Diekelmann S, Wilhelm I, Born J. The whats and whens of sleep-dependent memory consolidation. Sleep Med Rev. 2009 Oct;13(5):309-21

Ferrie JE, Shipley MJ, Akbaraly TN, Marmot MG, Kivimäki M, Singh-Manoux A. Change in sleep duration and cognitive function: findings from the Whitehall II Study. Sleep. 2011 May 1;34(5):565-73

Galli G, Piaggi P, Mattingly MS, de Jonge L, Courville AB, Pinchera A, Santini F, Csako G, Cizza G. Inverse relationship of food and alcohol intake to sleep measures in obesity. Nutr Diabetes. 2013 Jan 28;3:e58

Hairston KG, Bryer-Ash M, Norris JM, Haffner S, Bowden DW, Wagenknecht LE. Sleep duration and five-year abdominal fat accumulation in a minority cohort: the IRAS family study. Sleep. 2010 Mar;33(3):289-95

Heath G, Roach GD, Dorrian J, Ferguson SA, Darwent D, Sargent C. The effect of sleep restriction on snacking behaviour during a week of simulated shiftwork. Accid Anal Prev. 2012 Mar;45 Suppl:62-7

Johns MW. A new method for measuring daytime sleepiness: the Epworth sleepiness scale. Sleep. 1991 Dec;14(6):540-5

Kessler RC, Berglund PA, Coulouvrat C, Hajak G, Roth T, Shahly V, Shillington AC, Stephenson JJ, Walsh JK. Insomnia and the performance of US workers: results from the America insomnia survey. Sleep. 2011 Sep 1;34(9):1161-71

Knutson KL. Sleep duration and cardiometabolic risk: a review of the epidemiologic evidence. Best Pract Res Clin Endocrinol Metab. 2010 Oct;24(5):731-43

Knutson KL, Spiegel K, Penev P, Van Cauter E. The metabolic consequences of sleep deprivation. Sleep Med Rev. 2007 Jun;11(3):163-78

Léger D, Bayon V. Societal costs of insomnia. Sleep Med Rev. 2010 Dec;14(6):379-89

Littner MR, Kushida C, Wise M, Davila DG, Morgenthaler T, Lee-Chiong T, Hirshkowitz M, Daniel LL, Bailey D, Berry RB, Kapen S, Kramer M; Standards of Practice Committee of the American Academy of Sleep Medicine. Practice parameters for clinical use of the multiple sleep latency test and the maintenance of wakefulness test. Sleep. 2005 Jan;28(1):113-21

Markwald RR, Melanson EL, Smith MR, Higgins J, Perreault L, Eckel RH, Wright KP Jr. Impact of insufficient sleep on total daily energy expenditure, food intake, and weight gain. Proc Natl Acad Sci U S A. 2013 Apr 2;110(14):5695-700

Maruff P, Falleti MG, Collie A, Darby D, McStephen M. Fatigue-related impairment in the speed, accuracy and variability of psychomotor performance: comparison with blood alcohol levels. J Sleep Res. 2005 Mar;14(1):21-7

Morselli L, Leproult R, Balbo M, Spiegel K. Role of sleep duration in the regulation of glucose metabolism and appetite. Best Pract Res Clin Endocrinol Metab. 2010 Oct;24(5):687-702

Owens JA. Sleep loss and fatigue in healthcare professionals. J Perinat Neonatal Nurs. 2007 Apr-Jun;21(2):92-100

Parsai S. Examining the relationship between sleep and obesity using subjective and objective methods. 2011. Iowa State University graduate theses and dissertations

Patel SR. Reduced sleep as an obesity risk factor. Obes Rev. 2009 Nov;10 Suppl 2:61-8

Reynolds AC, Dorrian J, Liu PY, Van Dongen HP, Wittert GA, Harmer LJ, Banks S. Impact of five nights of sleep restriction on glucose metabolism, leptin and testosterone in young adult men. PLoS One. 2012;7(7):e41218

Schmid SM, Hallschmid M, Jauch-Chara K, Wilms B, Lehnert H, Born J, Schultes B. Disturbed glucoregulatory response to food intake after moderate sleep restriction. Sleep. 2011 Mar 1;34(3):371-7

Schoenborn CA, Adams PF. Sleep duration as a correlate of smoking, alcohol use, leisure-time physical inactivity, and obesity among adults: United States, 2004-2006. 2008:May. NCHS Health & Stats

Shatzmiller RA. Sleep Stage Scoring. Medcape Reference. 2010;Jun 17. http://emedicine.medscape.com/article/1188142-overview

Shlisky JD, Hartman TJ, Kris-Etherton PM, Rogers CJ, Sharkey NA, Nickols-Richardson SM. Partial sleep deprivation and energy balance in adults: an emerging issue for consideration by dietetics practitioners. J Acad Nutr Diet. 2012 Nov;112(11):1785-97

Spiegel K, Tasali E, Penev P, Van Cauter E. Brief communication: Sleep curtailment in healthy young men is associated with decreased leptin levels, elevated ghrelin levels, and increased hunger and appetite. Ann Intern Med. 2004 Dec 7;141(11):846-50

St-Onge MP. The role of sleep duration in the regulation of energy balance: effects on energy intakes and expenditure. J Clin Sleep Med. 2013 Jan 15;9(1):73-80

St-Onge MP, McReynolds A, Trivedi ZB, Roberts AL, Sy M, Hirsch J. Sleep restriction leads to increased activation of brain regions sensitive to food stimuli. Am J Clin Nutr. 2012 Apr;95(4):818-24

St-Onge MP, O'Keeffe M, Roberts AL, RoyChoudhury A, Laferrère B. Short sleep duration, glucose dysregulation and hormonal regulation of appetite in men and women. Sleep. 2012 Nov 1;35(11):1503-10

Taras H, Potts-Datema W. Sleep and student performance at school. J Sch Health. 2005 Sep;75(7):248-54

Valent F, Di Bartolomeo S, Marchetti R, Sbrojavacca R, Barbone F. A case-crossover study of sleep and work hours and the risk of road traffic accidents. Sleep. 2010 Mar;33(3):349-54

Vandekerckhove M, Cluydts R. The emotional brain and sleep: an intimate relationship. Sleep Med Rev. 2010 Aug;14(4):219-26

Walker MP. Sleep, memory and emotion. Prog Brain Res. 2010;185:49-68

Chapter 3: Reset the Body Clock

Brown GM. Light, melatonin and the sleep-wake cycle. J Psychiatry Neurosci. 1994 Nov;19(5):345-53

Cajochen C, Chellappa S, Schmidt C. What keeps us awake? The role of clocks and hourglasses, light, and melatonin. Int Rev Neurobiol. 2010;93:57-90

Campbell B, Wilborn C, La Bounty P, Taylor L, Nelson MT, Greenwood M, Ziegenfuss TN, Lopez HL, Hoffman JR, Stout JR, Schmitz S, Collins R, Kalman DS, Antonio J, Kreider RB. International Society of Sports Nutrition position stand: energy drinks. J Int Soc Sports Nutr. 2013 Jan 3;10(1):1

Duffy JF, Cain SW, Chang AM, Phillips AJ, Münch MY, Gronfier C, Wyatt JK, Dijk DJ, Wright KP Jr, Czeisler CA. Sex difference in the near-24-hour intrinsic period of the human circadian timing system. Proc Natl Acad Sci U S A. 2011 Sep 13;108 Suppl 3:15602-8

Food and Drug Administration. Caffeine intake by the US population. http://www.fda.gov/downloads/about FDA/CentersOffices/OfficeofFoods/CFSAN/CFSAN-FOIAElectronicReadingRoom/UCM333191.pdf

Froy O. Metabolism and circadian rhythms--implications for obesity. Endocr Rev. 2010 Feb;31(1):1-24

Giles GE, Mahoney CR, Brunyé TT, Gardony AL, Taylor HA, Kanarek RB. Differential cognitive effects of energy drink ingredients: caffeine, taurine, and glucose. Pharmacol Biochem Behav. 2012 Oct;102(4):569-77

Gooley JJ. Treatment of circadian rhythm sleep disorders with light. Ann Acad Med Singapore. 2008 Aug;37(8):669-76

Gooley JJ, Chamberlain K, Smith KA, Khalsa SB, Rajaratnam SM, Van Reen E, Zeitzer JM, Czeisler CA, Lockley SW. Exposure to room light before bedtime suppresses melatonin onset and shortens melatonin duration in humans. J Clin Endocrinol Metab. 2011 Mar;96(3):E463-72

Gordijn MC, 't Mannetje D, Meesters Y. The effects of blue-enriched light treatment compared to standard light treatment in Seasonal Affective Disorder. J Affect Disord. 2012 Jan;136(1-2):72-80

Highlights of changes from DSM-IV-TR to DSM-5. http://www.dsm5.org/Documents/changes%20from%20dsm-iv-tr%20to%20dsm-5.pdf

Hindmarch I, Rigney U, Stanley N, Quinlan P, Rycroft J, Lane J. A naturalistic investigation of the effects of day-long consumption of tea, coffee and water on alertness, sleep onset and sleep quality. Psychopharmacology (Berl). 2000 Apr;149(3):203-16

Hossain JL, Shapiro CM. Considerations and possible consequences of shift work. J Psychosom Res. 1999 Oct;47(4):293-6

Ishak WW, Ugochukwu C, Bagot K, Khalili D, Zaky C. Energy drinks: psychological effects and impact on well-being and quality of life-a literature review. Innov Clin Neurosci. 2012 Jan;9(1):25-34

James JE, Keane MA. Caffeine, sleep and wakefulness: implications of new understanding about withdrawal reversal. Hum Psychopharmacol. 2007 Dec;22(8):549-58

Lerman SE, Eskin E, Flower DJ, George EC, Gerson B, Hartenbaum N, Hursh SR, Moore-Ede M; American College of Occupational and Environmental Medicine Presidential Task Force on Fatigue Risk Management. Fatigue risk management in the workplace. J Occup Environ Med. 2012 Feb;54(2):231-58

Lucassen EA, Zhao X, Rother KI, Mattingly MS, Courville AB, de Jonge L, Csako G, Cizza G; Sleep Extension Study Group. Evening chronotype is associated with changes in eating behavior, more sleep apnea, and increased stress hormones in short sleeping obese individuals. PLoS One. 2013;8(3):e56519

Lurie SJ, Gawinski B, Pierce D, Rousseau SJ. Seasonal affective disorder. Am Fam Physician. 2006 Nov 1;74(9):1521-4

Maughan RJ, Griffin J. Caffeine ingestion and fluid balance: a review. J Hum Nutr Diet. 2003 Dec;16(6):411-20

McLellan TM, Lieberman HR. Do energy drinks contain active components other than caffeine? Nutr Rev. 2012 Dec;70(12):730-44

Münch M, Bromundt V. Light and chronobiology: implications for health and disease. Dialogues Clin Neurosci. 2012 Dec;14(4):448-53

Nehlig A. Is caffeine a cognitive enhancer? J Alzheimers Dis. 2010;20 Suppl 1:S85-94

Persad LA. Energy drinks and the neurophysiological impact of caffeine. Front Neurosci. 2011;5:116

Peuhkuri K, Sihvola N, Korpela R. Dietary factors and fluctuating levels of melatonin. Food Nutr Res. 2012;56

Roehrs T, Roth T. Caffeine: sleep and daytime sleepiness. Sleep Med Rev. 2008 Apr;12(2):153-62

Rosenthal NE. Diagnosis and treatment of seasonal affective disorder. JAMA. 1993 Dec 8;270(22):2717-20

Rüger M, Scheer FA. Effects of circadian disruption on the cardiometabolic system. Rev Endocr Metab Disord. 2009 Dec;10(4):245-60

Sack RL, Auckley D, Auger RR, Carskadon MA, Wright KP Jr, Vitiello MV, Zhdanova IV; American Academy of Sleep Medicine. Circadian rhythm sleep disorders: part I, basic principles, shift work and jet lag disorders. An American Academy of Sleep Medicine review. Sleep. 2007 Nov;30(11):1460-83

Santhi N, Aeschbach D, Horowitz TS, Czeisler CA. The impact of sleep timing and bright light exposure on attentional impairment during night work. J Biol Rhythms. 2008 Aug;23(4):341-52

Shen J, Botly LC, Chung SA, Gibbs AL, Sabanadzovic S, Shapiro CM. Fatigue and shift work. J Sleep Res. 2006 Mar;15(1):1-5

Smith AP. Caffeine at work. Hum Psychopharmacol. 2005 Aug;20(6):441-5

Smith AP. Caffeine, cognitive failures and health in a non-working community sample. Hum Psychopharmacol. 2009 Jan;24(1):29-34

Smith MR, Eastman CI. Shift work: health, performance and safety problems, traditional countermeasures, and innovative management strategies to reduce circadian misalignment. Nat Sci Sleep. 2012 Sep 27;4:111-32.

Snel J, Lorist MM. Effects of caffeine on sleep and cognition. Prog Brain Res. 2011;190:105-17

Takahashi M. Prioritizing sleep for healthy work schedules. J Physiol Anthropol. 2012 Mar 13;31:6

Terman M. Evolving applications of light therapy. Sleep Med Rev. 2007 Dec;11(6):497-507

Wang XS, Armstrong ME, Cairns BJ, Key TJ, Travis RC. Shift work and chronic disease: the epidemiological evidence. Occup Med (Lond). 2011 Mar;61(2):78-89

Waterhouse J, Fukuda Y, Morita T. Daily rhythms of the sleep-wake cycle. J Physiol Anthropol. 2012 Mar 13;31:5

Wright KP Jr, Gronfier C, Duffy JF, Czeisler CA. Intrinsic period and light intensity determine the phase relationship between melatonin and sleep in humans. J Biol Rhythms. 2005 Apr;20(2):168-77

Zeitzer JM, Dijk DJ, Kronauer R, Brown E, Czeisler C. Sensitivity of the human circadian pacemaker to nocturnal light: melatonin phase resetting and suppression. J Physiol. 2000 Aug 1;526 Pt 3:695-702

Chapter 4: Take Strategic Breaks

Ariga A, Lleras A. Brief and rare mental "breaks" keep you focused: deactivation and reactivation of task goals preempt vigilance decrements. Cognition. 2011 Mar;118(3):439-43

Campos H, Siles X. Siesta and the risk of coronary heart disease: results from a population-based, case-control study in Costa Rica. Int J Epidemiol. 2000 Jun;29(3):429-37

Danziger S, Levav J, Avnaim-Pesso L. Extraneous factors in judicial decisions. Proc Natl Acad Sci U S A. 2011 Apr 26;108(17):6889-92

Ficca G, Axelsson J, Mollicone DJ, Muto V, Vitiello MV. Naps, cognition and performance. Sleep Med Rev. 2010 Aug;14(4):249-58

Hays JC, Blazer DG, Foley DJ. Risk of napping: excessive daytime sleepiness and mortality in an older community population. J Am Geriatr Soc. 1996 Jun;44(6):693-8

Horne J, Anderson C, Platten C. Sleep extension versus nap or coffee, within the context of 'sleep debt'. J Sleep Res. 2008 Dec;17(4):432-6

Holmes A, Al-Bayat S, Hilditch C, Bourgeois-Bougrine S. Sleep and sleepiness during an ultra long-range flight operation between the Middle East and United States. Accid Anal Prev. 2012 Mar;45 Suppl:27-31

Kaida K, Takeda Y, Tsuzuki K. The relationship between flow, sleepiness and cognitive performance: the effects of short afternoon nap and bright light exposure. Ind Health. 2012;50(3):189-96

Lovato N, Lack L. The effects of napping on cognitive functioning. Prog Brain Res. 2010;185:155-66

Marcora SM, Staiano W, Manning V. Mental fatigue impairs physical performance in humans. J Appl Physiol (1985). 2009 Mar;106(3):857-64

Mednick SC, Cai DJ, Kanady J, Drummond SP. Comparing the benefits of caffeine, naps and placebo on verbal, motor and perceptual memory. Behav Brain Res. 2008 Nov 3;193(1):79-86

Mehra R, Patel SR. To nap or not to nap: that is the question. Sleep. 2012 Jul 1;35(7):903-4

Milner CE, Cote KA. Benefits of napping in healthy adults: impact of nap length, time of day, age, and experience with napping. J Sleep Res. 2009 Jun;18(2):272-81

Rosekind MR, Dinges DF, Connell LJ, Rountree MS, Spinweber CL, Gillen KA. Crew factors in flight operations IX: effects of planned cockpit rest on crew performance and alertness in long haul operations. 1994. Moffett Field, CA: NASA Ames Research Center. http://www.utu324.com/agreements/Union%20Docs/Fatigue%20Rest/FRF-008.pdf

Rosekind MR Gander PH, Connell LJ, Co EL. 2001. Crew factors in flight operations X: alertness management in flight operations education module. 2001. NASA. Ames Research Center. http://humanfactors.arc.nasa.gov/publications/ETM-X2001.pdf

Rosekind MR, Smith RM, Miller DL, Co EL, Gregory KB, Webbon LL, Gander PH, Lebacqz JV. Alertness management: strategic naps in operational settings. J Sleep Res. 1995 Dec;4(S2):62-66

Takahashi M. The role of prescribed napping in sleep medicine. Sleep Med Rev. 2003 Jun;7(3):227-35

Chapter 5: Listen to Your Body Talk (No, You're Not Crazy)

Ainsworth BE, Haskell WL, Herrmann SD, Meckes N, Bassett DR Jr, Tudor-Locke C, Greer JL, Vezina J, Whitt-Glover MC, Leon AS. 2011 Compendium of Physical Activities: a second update of codes and MET values. Med Sci Sports Exerc. 2011 Aug;43(8):1575-81

Andrade AM, Greene GW, Melanson KJ. Eating slowly led to decreases in energy intake within meals in healthy women. J Am Diet Assoc. 2008 Jul;108(7):1186-91

Benton D, Parker PY. Breakfast, blood glucose, and cognition. Am J Clin Nutr. 1998 Apr;67(4):772S-778S

Brunstrom JM. The control of meal size in human subjects: a role for expected satiety, expected satiation and premeal planning. Proc Nutr Soc. 2011 May;70(2):155-61

Cahill GF Jr. Starvation in man. Clin Endocrinol Metab. 1976 Jul;5(2):397-415

Campfield LA, Smith FJ. Blood glucose dynamics and control of meal initiation: a pattern detection and recognition theory. Physiol Rev. 2003 Jan;83(1):25-58

Chaplin K, Smith AP. Breakfast and snacks: associations with cognitive failures, minor injuries, accidents and stress. Nutrients. 2011 May;3(5):515-28

de Castro JM. The time of day of food intake influences overall intake in humans. J Nutr. 2004 Jan;134(1):104-11

Ello-Martin JA, Ledikwe JH, Rolls BJ. The influence of food portion size and energy density on energy intake: implications for weight management. Am J Clin Nutr. 2005 Jul;82(1 Suppl):236S-241S

Frankenfield D, Roth-Yousey L, Compher C. Comparison of predictive equations for resting metabolic rate in healthy nonobese and obese adults: a systematic review. J Am Diet Assoc. 2005 May;105(5):775-89

Gailliot MT, Baumeister RF, DeWall CN, Maner JK, Plant EA, Tice DM, Brewer LE, Schmeichel BJ. Self-control relies on glucose as a limited energy source: willpower is more than a metaphor. J Pers Soc Psychol. 2007 Feb;92(2):325-36

Gailliot MT, Baumeister RF. The physiology of willpower: linking blood glucose to self-control. Pers Soc Psychol Rev. 2007 Nov;11(4):303-27

Galgani J, Ravussin E. Energy metabolism, fuel selection and body weight regulation. Int J Obes (Lond). 2008 Dec;32 Suppl 7:S109-19

Goldstone AP, Prechtl de Hernandez CG, Beaver JD, Muhammed K, Croese C, Bell G, Durighel G, Hughes E, Waldman AD, Frost G, Bell JD. Fasting biases brain reward systems towards high-calorie foods. Eur J Neurosci. 2009 Oct;30(8):1625-35

Hall KD. Predicting metabolic adaptation, body weight change, and energy intake in humans. Am J Physiol Endocrinol Metab. 2010 Mar;298(3):E449-66

Hall KD, Sacks G, Chandramohan D, Chow CC, Wang YC, Gortmaker SL, Swinburn BA. Quantification of the effect of energy imbalance on bodyweight. Lancet. 2011 Aug 27;378(9793):826-37

Hogenkamp PS. Effect of oral processing behavior on food intake and satiety. Trends in Food Science & Technology. 2013 Sep.

Holt SH, Delargy HJ, Lawton CL, Blundell JE. The effects of high-carbohydrate vs high-fat breakfasts on feelings of fullness and alertness, and subsequent food intake. Int J Food Sci Nutr. 1999 Jan;50(1):13-28

Hoyland A, Dye L, Lawton CL. A systematic review of the effect of breakfast on the cognitive performance of children and adolescents. Nutr Res Rev. 2009 Dec;22(2):220-43

Jakubowicz D, Froy O, Wainstein J, Boaz M. Meal timing and composition influence ghrelin levels, appetite scores and weight loss maintenance in overweight and obese adults. Steroids. 2012 Mar 10;77(4):323-31

Janssen P, Vanden Berghe P, Verschueren S, Lehmann A, Depoortere I, Tack J. Review article: the role of gastric motility in the control of food intake. Aliment Pharmacol Ther. 2011 Apr;33(8):880-94

Jebb SA, Murgatroyd PR, Goldberg GR, Prentice AM, Coward WA. In vivo measurement of changes in body composition: description of methods and their validation against 12-d continuous whole-body calorimetry. Am J Clin Nutr. 1993 Oct;58(4):455-62

Jebb SA, Prentice AM, Goldberg GR, Murgatroyd PR, Black AE, Coward WA. Changes in macronutrient balance during over- and underfeeding assessed by 12-d continuous whole-body calorimetry. Am J Clin Nutr. 1996 Sep;64(3):259-66

Leidy HJ, Ortinau LC, Douglas SM, Hoertel HA. Beneficial effects of a higher-protein breakfast on the appetitive, hormonal, and neural signals controlling energy intake regulation in overweight/obese, "breakfast-skipping," late-adolescent girls. Am J Clin Nutr. 2013 Apr;97(4):677-88

Marchiori D, Waroquier L, Klein O. Smaller food item sizes of snack foods influence reduced portions and caloric intake in young adults. J Am Diet Assoc. 2011 May;111(5):727-31

McDevitt RM, Poppitt SD, Murgatroyd PR, Prentice AM. Macronutrient disposal during controlled overfeeding with glucose, fructose, sucrose, or fat in lean and obese women. Am J Clin Nutr. 2000 Aug;72(2):369-77

Meikle A, Riby LM, Stollery B. The impact of glucose ingestion and glucoregulatory control on cognitive performance: a comparison of younger and middle aged adults. Hum Psychopharmacol. 2004 Dec;19(8):523-35

Mekary RA, Giovannucci E, Willett WC, van Dam RM, Hu FB. Eating patterns and type 2 diabetes risk in men: breakfast omission, eating frequency, and snacking. Am J Clin Nutr. 2012 May;95(5):1182-9

Messier C. Glucose improvement of memory: a review. Eur J Pharmacol. 2004 Apr 19;490(1-3):33-57

Mifflin MD, St Jeor ST, Hill LA, Scott BJ, Daugherty SA, Koh YO. A new predictive equation for resting energy expenditure in healthy individuals. Am J Clin Nutr. 1990 Feb;51(2):241-7

Nabb S, Benton D. The influence on cognition of the interaction between the macro-nutrient content of breakfast and glucose tolerance. Physiol Behav. 2006 Jan 30;87(1):16-23

Otten JJ, Hellwig JP, & Meyers LD (eds). Dietary Reference Intakes: The Essential Guide to Nutrient Requirements (2006). The National Academies Press

Pereira MA, Erickson E, McKee P, Schrankler K, Raatz SK, Lytle LA, Pellegrini AD. Breakfast frequency and quality may affect glycemia and appetite in adults and children. J Nutr. 2011 Jan;141(1):163-8

Pivik RT, Tennal KB, Chapman SD, Gu Y. Eating breakfast enhances the efficiency of neural networks engaged during mental arithmetic in school-aged children. Physiol Behav. 2012 Jun 25;106(4):548-55

Rampersaud GC, Pereira MA, Girard BL, Adams J, Metzl JD. Breakfast habits, nutritional status, body weight, and academic performance in children and adolescents. J Am Diet Assoc. 2005 May;105(5):743-60

Redman LM, Heilbronn LK, Martin CK, Alfonso A, Smith SR, Ravussin E; Pennington CALERIE Team. Effect of calorie restriction with or without exercise on body composition and fat distribution. J Clin Endocrinol Metab. 2007 Mar;92(3):865-72

Rolls BJ. The role of energy density in the overconsumption of fat. J Nutr. 2000 Feb;130(2S Suppl):268S-271S

Rolls BJ, Roe LS, Meengs JS. Larger portion sizes lead to a sustained increase in energy intake over 2 days. J Am Diet Assoc. 2006 Apr;106(4):543-9

Ruijschop RM, Zijlstra N, Boelrijk AE, Dijkstra A, Burgering MJ, Graaf Cd, Westerterp-Plantenga MS. Effects of bite size and duration of oral processing on retro-nasal aroma release - features contributing to meal termination. Br J Nutr. 2011 Jan;105(2):307-15

Sacks FM, Bray GA, Carey VJ, Smith SR, Ryan DH, Anton SD, McManus K, Champagne CM, Bishop LM, Laranjo N, Leboff MS, Rood JC, de Jonge L, Greenway FL, Loria CM, Obarzanek E, Williamson DA. Comparison of weight-loss diets with different compositions of fat, protein, and carbohydrates. N Engl J Med. 2009 Feb 26;360(9):859-73

Shimizu M, Payne CR, Wansink B. When snacks become meals: How hunger and environmental cues bias food intake. Int J Behav Nutr Phys Act. 2010 Aug 25;7:63

Smeets AJ, Westerterp-Plantenga MS. Acute effects on metabolism and appetite profile of one meal difference in the lower range of meal frequency. Br J Nutr. 2008 Jun;99(6):1316-21

Solomon TP, Chambers ES, Jeukendrup AE, Toogood AA, Blannin AK. The effect of feeding frequency on insulin and ghrelin responses in human subjects. Br J Nutr. 2008 Oct;100(4):810-9

Stull AJ, Apolzan JW, Thalacker-Mercer AE, Iglay HB, Campbell WW. Liquid and solid meal replacement products differentially affect postprandial appetite and food intake in older adults. J Am Diet Assoc. 2008 Jul;108(7):1226-30

Thomas JG, Bond DS, Phelan S, Hill JO, Wing RR. Weight-loss maintenance for 10 years in the national weight control registry. Am J Prev Med. 2014 Jan;46(1):17-23

van der Heijden AA, Hu FB, Rimm EB, van Dam RM. A prospective study of breakfast consumption and weight gain among U.S. men. Obesity (Silver Spring). 2007 Oct;15(10):2463-9

Wansink B, Payne CR, Chandon P. Internal and external cues of meal cessation: the French paradox redux? Obesity (Silver Spring). 2007 Dec;15(12):2920-4

Wansink B, Tal A, Shimizu M. First foods most: after 18-hour fast, people drawn to starches first and vegetables last. Arch Intern Med. 2012 Jun 25;172(12):961-3

Wansink B, Payne CR, Shimizu M. The 100-calorie semi-solution: sub-packaging most reduces intake among the heaviest. Obesity (Silver Spring). 2011 May;19(5):1098-100

Wansink B, van Ittersum K. Portion size me: downsizing our consumption norms. J Am Diet Assoc. 2007 Jul;107(7):1103-6

Wells AS, Read NW. Influences of fat, energy, and time of day on mood and performance. Physiol Behav. 1996 Jun;59(6):1069-76

Westerterp KR. Physical activity and physical activity induced energy expenditure in humans: measurement, determinants, and effects. Front Physiol. 2013;4:90

Wing RR, Phelan S. Long-term weight loss maintenance. Am J Clin Nutr. 2005 Jul;82(1 Suppl):222S-225S

Chapter 6: Check Your Fuel Gauge

American Diabetes Association. Standards of medical care in diabetes--2014. Diabetes Care. 2014 Jan;37 Suppl 1:S14-80

Bock G, Dalla Man C, Campioni M, Chittilapilly E, Basu R, Toffolo G, Cobelli C, Rizza R. Pathogenesis of pre-diabetes: mechanisms of fasting and postprandial hyperglycemia in people with impaired fasting glucose and/or impaired glucose tolerance. Diabetes. 2006 Dec;55(12):3536-49

Ciampolini M, Bianchi R. Training to estimate blood glucose and to form associations with initial hunger. Nutr Metab (Lond). 2006 Dec 8;3:42

Davis SN, Shavers C, Costa F. Differential gender responses to hypoglycemia are due to alterations in CNS drive and not glycemic thresholds. Am J Physiol Endocrinol Metab. 2000 Nov;279(5):E1054-63

Fourest-Fontecave S, Adamson U, Lins PE, Ekblom B, Sandahl C, Strand L. Mental alertness in response to hypoglycaemia in normal man: the effect of 12 hours and 72 hours of fasting. Diabete Metab. 1987 Jul-Aug;13(4):405-10

Lucidi P, Rossetti P, Porcellati F, Pampanelli S, Candeloro P, Andreoli AM, Perriello G, Bolli GB, Fanelli CG. Mechanisms of insulin resistance after insulin-induced hypoglycemia in humans: the role of lipolysis. Diabetes. 2010 Jun;59(6):1349-57

Mellman MJ, Davis MR, Brisman M, Shamoon H. Effect of antecedent hypoglycemia on cognitive function and on glycemic thresholds for counterregulatory hormone secretion in healthy humans. Diabetes Care. 1994 Mar;17(3):183-8

Roach PJ. Glycogen and its metabolism. Curr Mol Med. 2002 Mar;2(2):101-20

Simpson EJ, Holdsworth M, Macdonald IA. Interstitial glucose profile associated with symptoms attributed to hypoglycemia by otherwise healthy women. Am J Clin Nutr. 2008 Feb;87(2):354-61

Taborsky GJ Jr. The physiology of glucagon. J Diabetes Sci Technol. 2010 Nov 1;4(6):1338-44

Tesfaye N, Seaquist ER. Neuroendocrine responses to hypoglycemia. Ann N Y Acad Sci. 2010 Nov;1212:12-28

Xu K, Morgan KT, Todd Gehris A, Elston TC, Gomez SM. A whole-body model for glycogen regulation reveals a critical role for substrate cycling in maintaining blood glucose homeostasis. PLoS Comput Biol. 2011 Dec;7(12):e1002272

Chapter 7: Refuel on a Regular Basis

Bachman JL, Phelan S, Wing RR, Raynor HA. Eating frequency is higher in weight loss maintainers and normal-weight individuals than in overweight individuals. J Am Diet Assoc. 2011 Nov;111(11):1730-4

Bachman JL, Raynor HA. Effects of manipulating eating frequency during a behavioral weight loss intervention: a pilot randomized controlled trial. Obesity (Silver Spring). 2012 May;20(5):985-92

Bes-Rastrollo M, Sanchez-Villegas A, Basterra-Gortari FJ, Nunez-Cordoba JM, Toledo E, Serrano-Martinez M. Prospective study of self-reported usual snacking and weight gain in a Mediterranean cohort: the SUN project. Clin Nutr. 2010 Jun;29(3):323-30

Cameron JD, Cyr MJ, Doucet E. Increased meal frequency does not promote greater weight loss in subjects who were prescribed an 8-week equi-energetic energy-restricted diet. Br J Nutr. 2010;103:1098-1101.

Centers for Disease Control and Prevention. Prevalence of Overweight, Obesity, and Extreme Obesity Among Adults: United States, Trends 1960–1962 Through

2007–2008. http://www.cdc.gov/nchs/data/hestat/obesity_adult_07_08/obesity_adult_07_08.htm

Chapelot D. The role of snacking in energy balance: a biobehavioral approach. J Nutr. 2011 Jan;141(1):158-62

Chapelot D, Marmonier C, Aubert R, Allègre C, Gausseres N, Fantino M, Louis-Sylvestre J. Consequence of omitting or adding a meal in man on body composition, food intake, and metabolism. Obesity (Silver Spring). 2006 Feb;14(2):215-27

Clark EN, Dewey AM, Temple JL. Effects of daily snack food intake on food reinforcement depend on body mass index and energy density. Am J Clin Nutr. 2010 Feb;91(2):300-8

Craig A. Acute effects of meals on perceptual and cognitive efficiency. Nutr Rev. 1986 May;44 Suppl:163-71

Duval K, Strychar I, Cyr MJ, Prud'homme D, Rabasa-Lhoret R, Doucet E. Physical activity is a confounding factor of the relation between eating frequency and body composition. Am J Clin Nutr. 2008 Nov;88(5):1200-5

Deutz RC, Benardot D, Martin DE, Cody MM. Relationship between energy deficits and body composition in elite female gymnasts and runners. Med Sci Sports Exerc. 2000 Mar;32(3):659-68

Fábry P, Tepperman J. Meal frequency--a possible factor in human pathology. Am J Clin Nutr. 1970 Aug;23(8):1059-68

Gailliot MT, Baumeister RF. The physiology of willpower: linking blood glucose to self-control. Pers Soc Psychol Rev. 2007 Nov;11(4):303-27

Garaulet M, Gómez-Abellán P, Alburquerque-Béjar JJ, Lee YC, Ordovás JM, Scheer FA. Timing of food intake predicts weight loss effectiveness. Int J Obes (Lond). 2013 Apr;37(4):604-11. Erratum in: Int J Obes (Lond). 2013 Apr;37(4):624

Kirk TR. Role of dietary carbohydrate and frequent eating in body-weight control. Proc Nutr Soc. 2000 Aug;59(3):349-58.

La Bounty PM, Campbell BI, Wilson J, Galvan E, Berardi J, Kleiner SM, Kreider RB, Stout JR, Ziegenfuss T, Spano M, Smith A, Antonio J. International Society of Sports Nutrition position stand: meal frequency. J Int Soc Sports Nutr. 2011 Mar 16;8:4

Leidy HJ, Armstrong CL, Tang M, Mattes RD, Campbell WW. The influence of higher protein intake and greater eating frequency on appetite control in overweight and obese men. Obesity (Silver Spring). 2010 Sep;18(9):1725-32

Leidy HJ, Campbell WW. The effect of eating frequency on appetite control and food intake: brief synopsis of controlled feeding studies. J Nutr. 2011 Jan;141(1):154-7

Lichtman SW, Pisarska K, Berman ER, Pestone M, Dowling H, Offenbacher E, Weisel H, Heshka S, Matthews DE, Heymsfield SB. Discrepancy between self-reported and actual caloric intake and exercise in obese subjects. N Engl J Med. 1992 Dec 31;327(27):1893-8

Ma Y, Bertone ER, Stanek EJ 3rd, Reed GW, Hebert JR, Cohen NL, Merriam PA, Ockene IS. Association between eating patterns and obesity in a free-living US adult population. Am J Epidemiol. 2003 Jul 1;158(1):85-92

Marmonier C, Chapelot D, Fantino M, Louis-Sylvestre J. Snacks consumed in a nonhungry state have poor satiating efficiency: influence of snack composition on substrate utilization and hunger. Am J Clin Nutr. 2002 Sep;76(3):518-28

McCrory MA, Howarth NC, Roberts SB, Huang TT. Eating frequency and energy regulation in free-living adults consuming self-selected diets. J Nutr. 2011 Jan;141(1):148-53

McCrory MA, Campbell WW. Effects of eating frequency, snacking, and breakfast skipping on energy regulation: symposium overview. J Nutr. 2011 Jan;141(1):144-7

Mills JP, Perry CD, Reicks M. Eating frequency is associated with energy intake but not obesity in midlife women. Obesity (Silver Spring). 2011 Mar;19(3):552-9

Piernas C, Popkin BM. Snacking increased among U.S. adults between 1977 and 2006. J Nutr. 2010 Feb;140(2):325-32

Rashidi MR, Mahboob S, Sattarivand R. Effects of nibbling and gorging on lipid profiles, blood glucose and insulin levels in healthy subjects. Saudi Med J. 2003 Sep;24(9):945-8

Solomon TP, Chambers ES, Jeukendrup AE, Toogood AA, Blannin AK. The effect of feeding frequency on insulin and ghrelin responses in human subjects. Br J Nutr. 2008 Oct;100(4):810-9

Stroebele N, Ogden LG, Hill JO. Do calorie-controlled portion sizes of snacks reduce energy intake? Appetite. 2009 Jun;52(3):793-6

van Kleef E, Shimizu M, Wansink B. Just a bite: considerably smaller snack portions satisfy delayed hunger and craving. Food Quality & Preference. 2013 27:96-100

Yannakoulia M, Melistas L, Solomou E, Yiannakouris N. Association of eating frequency with body fatness in pre- and postmenopausal women. Obesity (Silver Spring). 2007 Jan;15(1):100-6

Chapter 8: Consider the Fuel Mix (aka What's On Your Plate)

Bohé J, Low A, Wolfe RR, Rennie MJ. Human muscle protein synthesis is modulated by extracellular, not intramuscular amino acid availability: a dose-response study. J Physiol. 2003 Oct 1;552(Pt 1):315-24

Brand-Miller JC, Holt SH, Pawlak DB, McMillan J. Glycemic index and obesity. Am J Clin Nutr 2002;76(1):281S-5S

Brand-Miller J, McMillan-Price J, Steinbeck K, Caterson I. Dietary glycemic index: health implications. J Am Coll Nutr. 2009 Aug;28 Suppl:446S-449S

Bray GA, Smith SR, DeJonge L, de Souza R, Rood J, Champagne CM, Laranjo N, Carey V, Obarzanek E, Loria CM, Anton SD, Ryan DH, Greenway FL, Williamson D, Sacks FM. Effect of diet composition on energy expenditure during weight loss: the POUNDS LOST Study. Int J Obes (Lond). 2012 Mar;36(3):448-55

Ebbeling CB, Swain JF, Feldman HA, Wong WW, Hachey DL, Garcia-Lago E, Ludwig DS. Effects of dietary composition on energy expenditure during weight-loss maintenance. JAMA. 2012 Jun 27;307(24):2627-34

Esfahani A, Wong JM, Mirrahimi A, Srichaikul K, Jenkins DJ, Kendall CW. The glycemic index: physiological significance. J Am Coll Nutr. 2009 Aug;28 Suppl:439S-445S

Foster-Powell K, Holt SH, Brand-Miller JC. International table of glycemic index and glycemic load values: 2002. Am J Clin Nutr. 2002 Jul;76(1):5-56

Galgani J, Aguirre C, Díaz E. Acute effect of meal glycemic index and glycemic load on blood glucose and insulin responses in humans. Nutr J. 2006 Sep 5;5:22

Gosby AK, Conigrave AD, Lau NS, Iglesias MA, Hall RM, Jebb SA, Brand-Miller J, Caterson ID, Raubenheimer D, Simpson SJ. Testing protein leverage in lean humans: a randomised controlled experimental study. PLoS One. 2011;6(10):e25929

Halton TL, Hu FB. The effects of high protein diets on thermogenesis, satiety and weight loss: a critical review. J Am Coll Nutr. 2004 Oct;23(5):373-85

Hession M, Rolland C, Kulkarni U, Wise A, Broom J. Systematic review of randomized controlled trials of low-carbohydrate vs. low-fat/low-calorie diets in the management of obesity and its comorbidities. Obes Rev. 2009 Jan;10(1):36-50

Jenkins DJ, Kendall CW, Augustin LS, Franceschi S, Hamidi M, Marchie A, Jenkins AL, Axelsen M. Glycemic index: overview of implications in health and disease. Am J Clin Nutr. 2002 Jul;76(1):266S-73S

Kreitzman SN, Coxon AY, Szaz KF. Glycogen storage: illusions of easy weight loss, excessive weight regain, and distortions in estimates of body composition. Am J Clin Nutr. 1992 Jul;56(1 Suppl):292S-293S

Lagerpusch M, Enderle J, Eggeling B, Braun W, Johannsen M, Pape D, Müller MJ, Bosy-Westphal A. Carbohydrate quality and quantity affect glucose and lipid metabolism during weight regain in healthy men. J Nutr. 2013 Oct;143(10):1593-601

Leidy HJ, Lepping RJ, Savage CR, Harris CT. Neural responses to visual food stimuli after a normal vs. higher protein breakfast in breakfast-skipping teens: a pilot fMRI study. Obesity (Silver Spring). 2011 Oct;19(10):2019-25

Leidy HJ, Mattes RD, Campbell WW. Effects of acute and chronic protein intake on metabolism, appetite, and ghrelin during weight loss. Obesity (Silver Spring). 2007 May;15(5):1215-25

Livesey G, Taylor R, Hulshof T, Howlett J. Glycemic response and health--a systematic review and meta-analysis: the database, study characteristics, and macronutrient intakes. Am J Clin Nutr. 2008 Jan;87(1):223S-236S

Lopes da Silva MV, de Càssia Gonçalves Alfenas R. Effect of the glycemic index on lipid oxidation and body composition. Nutr Hosp. 2011 Jan-Feb;26(1):48-55

Ludwig DS, Majzoub JA, Al-Zahrani A, Dallal GE, Blanco I, Roberts SB. High glycemic index foods, overeating, and obesity. Pediatrics. 1999 Mar;103(3):E26

Ma Y, Olendzki B, Chiriboga D, Hebert JR, Li Y, Li W, Campbell M, Gendreau K, Ockene IS. Association between dietary carbohydrates and body weight. Am J Epidemiol. 2005 Feb 15;161(4):359-67

Mamerow MM, Mettler JA, English KL, Casperson SL, Arentson-Lantz E, Sheffield-Moore M, Layman DK, Paddon-Jones D. Dietary protein distribution positively influences 24-h muscle protein synthesis in healthy adults. J Nutr. 2014 Jun;144(6):876-80

Marsh K, Brand-Miller J. State of the Art Reviews: Glycemic Index, Obesity, and Chronic Disease. Am J Lifestyle Med. 2008 Mar/Apr;2(2):142-150

Paddon-Jones D, Westman E, Mattes RD, Wolfe RR, Astrup A, Westerterp-Plantenga M. Protein, weight management, and satiety. Am J Clin Nutr. 2008 May;87(5):1558S-1561S

Phillips SM, Van Loon LJ. Dietary protein for athletes: from requirements to optimum adaptation. J Sports Sci. 2011;29 Suppl 1:S29-38

Santesso N, Akl EA, Bianchi M, Mente A, Mustafa R, Heels-Ansdell D, Schünemann HJ. Effects of higher- versus lower-protein diets on health outcomes: a systematic review and meta-analysis. Eur J Clin Nutr. 2012 Jul;66(7):780-8

Soenen S, Martens EA, Hochstenbach-Waelen A, Lemmens SG, Westerterp-Plantenga MS. Normal protein intake is required for body weight loss and weight maintenance, and elevated protein intake for additional preservation of resting energy expenditure and fat free mass. J Nutr. 2013 May;143(5):591-6

Sofer S, Eliraz A, Kaplan S, Voet H, Fink G, Kima T, Madar Z. Greater weight loss and hormonal changes after 6 months diet with carbohydrates eaten mostly at dinner. Obesity (Silver Spring). 2011 Oct;19(10):2006-14

Symons TB, Sheffield-Moore M, Wolfe RR, Paddon-Jones D. Moderating the portion size of a protein-rich meal improves anabolic efficiency in young and elderly. J Am Diet Assoc. 2009 Sept;109(9):1582-1586

Vega-López S, Ausman LM, Griffith JL, Lichtenstein AH. Interindividual variability and intra-individual reproducibility of glycemic index values for commercial white bread. Diabetes Care. 2007 Jun;30(6):1412-7

Weigle DS, Breen PA, Matthys CC, Callahan HS, Meeuws KE, Burden VR, Purnell JQ. A high-protein diet induces sustained reductions in appetite, ad libitum caloric intake, and body weight despite compensatory changes in diurnal plasma leptin and ghrelin concentrations. Am J Clin Nutr. 2005 Jul;82(1):41-8

Westerterp-Plantenga MS, Lejeune MP, Nijs I, van Ooijen M, Kovacs EM. High protein intake sustains weight maintenance after body weight loss in humans. Int J Obes Relat Metab Disord. 2004 Jan;28(1):57-64

Westerterp-Plantenga MS, Lemmens SG, Westerterp KR. Dietary protein - its role in satiety, energetics, weight loss and health. Br J Nutr. 2012 Aug;108 Suppl 2:S105-12

Westerterp-Plantenga MS, Nieuwenhuizen A, Tomé D, Soenen S, Westerterp KR. Dietary protein, weight loss, and weight maintenance. Annu Rev Nutr. 2009;29:21-41

Wycherley TP, Moran LJ, Clifton PM, Noakes M, Brinkworth GD. Effects of energy-restricted high-protein, low-fat compared with standard-protein, low-fat diets: a meta-analysis of randomized controlled trials. Am J Clin Nutr. 2012 Dec;96(6):1281-98

Chapter 9: Check the Fluid Level and Energy Boosters

Adan A. Cognitive performance and dehydration. J Am Coll Nutr. 2012 Apr;31(2):71-8

Alexander DD, Weed DL, Chang ET, Miller PE, Mohamed MA, Elkayam L. A systematic review of multivitamin-multimineral use and cardiovascular disease and cancer incidence and total mortality. J Am Coll Nutr. 2013;32(5):339-54

Armstrong LE, Ganio MS, Casa DJ, Lee EC, McDermott BP, Klau JF, Jimenez L, Le Bellego L, Chevillotte E, Lieberman HR. Mild dehydration affects mood in healthy young women. J Nutr. 2012 Feb;142(2):382-8

Bjelakovic G, Nikolova D, Gluud LL, Simonetti RG, Gluud C. Antioxidant supplements for prevention of mortality in healthy participants and patients with various diseases. Cochrane Database Syst Rev. 2012 Mar 14;3:CD007176

Burdon CA, Johnson NA, Chapman PG, O'Connor HT. Influence of beverage temperature on palatability and fluid ingestion during endurance exercise: a systematic review. Int J Sport Nutr Exerc Metab. 2012 Jun;22(3):199-211

Ganio MS, Armstrong LE, Casa DJ, McDermott BP, Lee EC, Yamamoto LM, Marzano S, Lopez RM, Jimenez L, Le Bellego L, Chevillotte E, Lieberman HR. Mild dehydration impairs cognitive performance and mood of men. Br J Nutr. 2011 Nov;106(10):1535-43

Gaziano JM, Glynn RJ, Christen WG, Kurth T, Belanger C, MacFadyen J, Bubes V, Manson JE, Sesso HD, Buring JE. Vitamins E and C in the prevention of prostate and total cancer in men: the Physicians' Health Study II randomized controlled trial. JAMA. 2009 Jan 7;301(1):52-62

Goodman GE, Thornquist MD, Balmes J, Cullen MR, Meyskens FL Jr, Omenn GS, Valanis B, Williams JH Jr. The Beta-Carotene and Retinol Efficacy Trial: incidence of lung cancer and cardiovascular disease mortality during 6-year follow-up after stopping beta-carotene and retinol supplements. J Natl Cancer Inst. 2004 Dec 1;96(23):1743-50

Grodstein F, O'Brien J, Kang JH, Dushkes R, Cook NR, Okereke O, Manson JE, Glynn RJ, Buring JE, Gaziano JM, Sesso HD. Long-term multivitamin supplementation and cognitive function in men: a randomized trial. Ann Intern Med. 2013 Dec;159(12):806-814

Institute of Medicine. Dietary reference intakes: water, potassium, sodium, chloride, and sulfate. 2004; Feb 11

Judelson DA, Maresh CM, Anderson JM, Armstrong LE, Casa DJ, Kraemer WJ, Volek JS. Hydration and muscular performance: does fluid balance affect strength, power and high-intensity endurance? Sports Med. 2007;37(10):907-21

Lafata D, Carlson-Phillips A, Sims ST, Russell EM. The effect of a cold beverage during an exercise session combining both strength and energy systems development training on core temperature and markers of performance. J Int Soc Sports Nutr. 2012 Sep 19;9(1):44

Lamas GA, Boineau R, Goertz C, Mark DB, Rosenberg Y, Stylianou M, Rozema T, Nahin RL, Lindblad L, Lewis EF, Drisko J, Lee KL. Oral high-dose multivitamins and minerals after myocardial infarction: a randomized trial. Ann Intern Med. 2013 Dec;159(12):797-805

Macpherson H, Pipingas A, Pase MP. Multivitamin-multimineral supplementation and mortality: a meta-analysis of randomized controlled trials. Am J Clin Nutr. 2013 Feb;97(2):437-44

Maughan RJ. Impact of mild dehydration on wellness and on exercise performance. Eur J Clin Nutr. 2003 Dec;57 Suppl 2:S19-23

Murray B. Hydration and physical performance. J Am Coll Nutr. 2007 Oct;26(5 Suppl):542S-548S

Neuhouser ML, Wassertheil-Smoller S, Thomson C, Aragaki A, Anderson GL, Manson JE, Patterson RE, Rohan TE, van Horn L, Shikany JM, Thomas A, LaCroix A, Prentice RL. Multivitamin use and risk of cancer and cardiovascular disease in the Women's Health Initiative cohorts. Arch Intern Med. 2009 Feb 9;169(3):294-304

Papaioannou D, Cooper KL, Carroll C, Hind D, Squires H, Tappenden P, Logan RF. Antioxidants in the chemoprevention of colorectal cancer and colorectal adenomas in the general population: a systematic review and meta-analysis. Colorectal Dis. 2011 Oct;13(10):1085-99

Reid ME, Duffield-Lillico AJ, Sunga A, Fakih M, Alberts DS, Marshall JR. Selenium supplementation and colorectal adenomas: an analysis of the nutritional prevention of cancer trial. Int J Cancer. 2006 Apr 1;118(7):1777-81

Shirreffs SM, Merson SJ, Fraser SM, Archer DT. The effects of fluid restriction on hydration status and subjective feelings in man. Br J Nutr. 2004 Jun;91(6):951-8

Stephen P. Fortmann, Brittany U. Burda, Caitlyn A. Senger, Jennifer S. Lin, Evelyn P. Whitlock; Vitamin and Mineral Supplements in the Primary Prevention of Cardiovascular Disease and Cancer: An Updated Systematic Evidence Review for the U.S. Preventive Services Task Force. Ann Intern Med. 2013 Dec;159(12):824-834

Szinnai G, Schachinger H, Arnaud MJ, Linder L, Keller U. Effect of water deprivation on cognitive-motor performance in healthy men and women. Am J Physiol Regul Integr Comp Physiol. 2005 Jul;289(1):R275-80

Wilk B, Rivera-Brown AM, Bar-Or O. Voluntary drinking and hydration in non-acclimatized girls exercising in the heat. Eur J Appl Physiol. 2007 Dec;101(6):727-34

Chapter 10: Eat What You Love

Afaghi A, O'Connor H, Chow CM. High-glycemic-index carbohydrate meals shorten sleep onset. Am J Clin Nutr. 2007 Feb;85(2):426-30. Erratum in: Am J Clin Nutr. 2007 Sep;86(3):809

Bellisle F, Drewnowski A. Intense sweeteners, energy intake and the control of body weight. Eur J Clin Nutr. 2007 Jun;61(6):691-700

Bellisle F, Drewnowski A, Anderson GH, Westerterp-Plantenga M, Martin CK. Sweetness, satiation, and satiety. J Nutr. 2012 Jun;142(6):1149S-54S

Byerley LO, Lee WN. Are ethanol and fructose similar? J Am Diet Assoc. 2010 Sep;110(9):1300-1

Caton SJ, Bate L, Hetherington MM. Acute effects of an alcoholic drink on food intake: aperitif versus co-ingestion. Physiol Behav. 2007 Feb 28;90(2-3):368-75

Fagherazzi G, Vilier A, Saes Sartorelli D, Lajous M, Balkau B, Clavel-Chapelon F. Consumption of artificially and sugar-sweetened beverages and incident type 2 diabetes in the Etude Epidemiologique aupres des femmes de la Mutuelle Generale de l'Education Nationale-European Prospective Investigation into Cancer and Nutrition cohort. Am J Clin Nutr. 2013 Mar;97(3):517-23

Figlewicz DP, Ioannou G, Bennett Jay J, Kittleson S, Savard C, Roth CL. Effect of moderate intake of sweeteners on metabolic health in the rat. Physiol Behav. 2009 Dec 7;98(5):618-24. Erratum in: Physiol Behav. 2010 Apr 19;99(5):691

Fitch C, Keim KS; Academy of Nutrition and Dietetics. Position of the Academy of Nutrition and Dietetics: use of nutritive and nonnutritive sweeteners. J Acad Nutr Diet. 2012 May;112(5):739-58. Erratum in: J Acad Nutr Diet. 2012 Aug;112(8):1279

Fowler SP, Williams K, Resendez RG, Hunt KJ, Hazuda HP, Stern MP. Fueling the obesity epidemic? Artificially sweetened beverage use and long-term weight gain. Obesity (Silver Spring). 2008 Aug;16(8):1894-900

Gardner C, Wylie-Rosett J, Gidding SS, Steffen LM, Johnson RK, Reader D, Lichtenstein AH; American Heart Association Nutrition Committee of the Council on Nutrition, Physical Activity and Metabolism, Council on Arteriosclerosis, Thrombosis and Vascular Biology, Council on Cardiovascular Disease in the Young; American Diabetes Association. Nonnutritive sweeteners: current use and health perspectives: a scientific statement from the American Heart Association and the American Diabetes Association. Diabetes Care. 2012 Aug;35(8):1798-808

Irwin C, Leveritt M, Shum D, Desbrow B. The effects of dehydration, moderate alcohol consumption, and rehydration on cognitive functions. Alcohol. 2013 May;47(3):203-13

Johnson RK, Appel LJ, Brands M, Howard BV, Lefevre M, Lustig RH, Sacks F, Steffen LM, Wylie-Rosett J. Dietary sugars intake and cardiovascular health: A scientific statement from the American Heart Association. Circ. 2009;120:1011-1020

Lustig RH. Fructose: metabolic, hedonic, and societal parallels with ethanol. J Am Diet Assoc. 2010 Sep;110(9):1307-21

Moubarac JC, Cargo M, Receveur O, Daniel M. Psychological distress mediates the association between daytime sleepiness and consumption of sweetened products: cross-sectional findings in a Catholic Middle-Eastern Canadian community. BMJ Open. 2013 Feb 13;3(2)

Rolls BJ. Effects of intense sweeteners on hunger, food intake, and body weight: a review. Am J Clin Nutr. 1991 Apr;53(4):872-8

Scholey A, Owen L. Effects of chocolate on cognitive function and mood: a systematic review. Nutr Rev. 2013 Oct;71(10):665-81

Sun SZ, Empie MW. Fructose metabolism in humans - what isotopic tracer studies tell us. Nutr Metab (Lond). 2012 Oct 2;9(1):89

Tappy L, Lê KA. Metabolic effects of fructose and the worldwide increase in obesity. Physiol Rev. 2010 Jan;90(1):23-46

Tappy L, Lê KA, Tran C, Paquot N. Fructose and metabolic diseases: new findings, new questions. Nutrition. 2010 Nov-Dec;26(11-12):1044-9

Tate DF, Turner-McGrievy G, Lyons E, Stevens J, Erickson K, Polzien K, Diamond M, Wang X, Popkin B. Replacing caloric beverages with water or diet beverages for weight loss in adults: main results of the Choose Healthy Options Consciously Everyday (CHOICE) randomized clinical trial. Am J Clin Nutr. 2012 Mar;95(3):555-63

Vannice G, Rasmussen H. Position of the academy of nutrition and dietetics: dietary Fatty acids for healthy adults. J Acad Nutr Diet. 2014 Jan;114(1):136-53

Vasdev S, Gill V, Singal PK. Beneficial effect of low ethanol intake on the cardiovascular system: possible biochemical mechanisms. Vasc Health Risk Manag. 2006;2(3):263-76

White JS. Straight talk about high-fructose corn syrup: what it is and what it ain't. Am J Clin Nutr. 2008 Dec;88(6):1716S-1721S

White JW, Wolraich M. Effect of sugar on behavior and mental performance. Am J Clin Nutr. 1995 Jul;62(1 Suppl):242S-247S

Yang Q. Gain weight by "going diet?" Artificial sweeteners and the neurobiology of sugar cravings: Neuroscience 2010. Yale J Biol Med. 2010 Jun;83(2):101-8

Yeomans MR. Alcohol, appetite and energy balance: is alcohol intake a risk factor for obesity? Physiol Behav. 2010 Apr 26;100(1):82-9

Chapter 11: Break the Stress Cycle

Andrea H, Beurskens AJ, Kant I, Davey GC, Field AP, van Schayck CP. The relation between pathological worrying and fatigue in a working population. J Psychosom Res. 2004 Oct;57(4):399-407

Boyle PA, Barnes LL, Buchman AS, Bennett DA. Purpose in life is associated with mortality among community-dwelling older persons. Psychosom Med. 2009 Jun;71(5):574-9

Carrasco GA, Van de Kar LD. Neuroendocrine pharmacology of stress. Eur J Pharmacol. 2003 Feb 28;463(1-3):235-72

Chida Y, Steptoe A. Positive psychological well-being and mortality: a quantitative review of prospective observational studies. Psychosom Med. 2008 Sep;70(7):741-56

Dean D, Webb C. Recovering from information overload. McKinsey Quarterly. 2011; Jan. Retrieved from http://www.mckinsey.com/insights/organization/recovering_from_information_overload on Feb 10, 2014

Epel E, Lapidus R, McEwen B, Brownell K. Stress may add bite to appetite in women: a laboratory study of stress-induced cortisol and eating behavior. Psychoneuroendocrinology. 2001 Jan;26(1):37-49

Epel ES, McEwen B, Seeman T, Matthews K, Castellazzo G, Brownell KD, Bell J, Ickovics JR. Stress and body shape: stress-induced cortisol secretion is consistently greater among women with central fat. Psychosom Med. 2000 Sep-Oct;62(5):623-32

Fortney L, Taylor M. Meditation in medical practice: a review of the evidence and practice. Prim Care. 2010 Mar;37(1):81-90

Goyal M, Singh S, Sibinga EM, Gould NF, Rowland-Seymour A, Sharma R, Berger Z, Sleicher D, Maron DD, Shihab HM, Ranasinghe PD, Linn S, Saha S, Bass EB, Haythornthwaite JA. Meditation Programs for Psychological Stress and Well-being: A Systematic Review and Meta-analysis. JAMA Intern Med. 2014 Jan 6

Law AS, Logie RH, Pearson DG. The impact of secondary tasks on multi-tasking in a virtual environment. Acta Psychol (Amst). 2006 May;122(1):27-44

Leary MR, Tate EB, Adams CE, Allen AB, Hancock J. Self-compassion and reactions to unpleasant self-relevant events: the implications of treating oneself kindly. J Pers Soc Psychol. 2007 May;92(5):887-904

McEwen BS. Physiology and neurobiology of stress and adaptation: central role of the brain. Physiol Rev. 2007 Jul;87(3):873-904

McEwen BS. The neurobiology of stress: from serendipity to clinical relevance. Brain Res. 2000 Dec 15;886(1-2):172-189

McEwen BS, Gianaros PJ. Central role of the brain in stress and adaptation: links to socioeconomic status, health, and disease. Ann N Y Acad Sci. 2010 Feb;1186:190-222

Rabito MJ, Kaye AD. Complementary and alternative medicine and cardiovascular disease: an evidence-based review. Evid Based Complement Alternat Med. 2013;2013:672097

Rosengren A, Hawken S, Ounpuu S, Sliwa K, Zubaid M, Almahmeed WA, Blackett KN, Sitthi-amorn C, Sato H, Yusuf S; INTERHEART investigators. Association of psychosocial risk factors with risk of acute myocardial infarction in 11119 cases and 13648 controls from 52 countries (the INTERHEART study): case-control study. Lancet. 2004 Sep 11-17;364(9438):953-62

Schaefer SM, Morozink Boylan J, van Reekum CM, Lapate RC, Norris CJ, Ryff CD, Davidson RJ. Purpose in life predicts better emotional recovery from negative stimuli. PLoS One. 2013 Nov 13;8(11):e80329

Snir R, Harpaz I. Beyond workaholism: Towards a general model of heavy work investment. Human Resource Mana Review (Impact Factor: 2.38). 09/2012; 22(3):232–243

Tang YY, Posner MI, Rothbart MK. Meditation improves self-regulation over the life span. Ann N Y Acad Sci. 2014 Jan;1307:104-11

Watkins ER. Constructive and unconstructive repetitive thought. Psychol Bull. 2008 Mar;134(2):163-206

Winbush NY, Gross CR, Kreitzer MJ. The effects of mindfulness-based stress reduction on sleep disturbance: a systematic review. Explore (NY). 2007 Nov-Dec;3(6):585-91

Chapter 12: Movement for Fun, Fitness, and Energy

Ahlskog JE, Geda YE, Graff-Radford NR, Petersen RC. Physical exercise as a preventive or disease-modifying treatment of dementia and brain aging. Mayo Clin Proc. 2011 Sep;86(9):876-84

American Dietetic Association; Dietitians of Canada; American College of Sports Medicine, Rodriguez NR, Di Marco NM, Langley S. American College of Sports Medicine position stand. Nutrition and athletic performance. Med Sci Sports Exerc. 2009 Mar;41(3):709-31

Blundell JE, Stubbs RJ, Hughes DA, Whybrow S, King NA. Cross talk between physical activity and appetite control: does physical activity stimulate appetite? Proc Nutr Soc. 2003 Aug;62(3):651-61

Chau JY, Grunseit AC, Chey T, Stamatakis E, Brown WJ, Matthews CE, Bauman AE, van der Ploeg HP. Daily sitting time and all-cause mortality: a meta-analysis. PLoS One. 2013;8(11):e80000

Chau JY, Grunseit A, Midthjell K, Holmen J, Holmen TL, Bauman AE, van der Ploeg HP. Cross-sectional associations of total sitting and leisure screen time with cardiometabolic risk in adults. Results from the HUNT Study, Norway. J Sci Med Sport. 2014 Jan;17(1):78-84

Colberg SR, Zarrabi L, Bennington L, Nakave A, Thomas Somma C, Swain DP, Sechrist SR. Postprandial walking is better for lowering the glycemic effect of dinner than pre-dinner exercise in type 2 diabetic individuals. J Am Med Dir Assoc. 2009 Jul;10(6):394-7

Fan JX, Brown BB, Hanson H, Kowaleski-Jones L, Smith KR, Zick CD. Moderate to vigorous physical activity and weight outcomes: does every minute count? Am J Health Promot. 2013 Sep-Oct;28(1):41-9

Garber CE, Blissmer B, Deschenes MR, Franklin BA, Lamonte MJ, Lee IM, Nieman DC, Swain DP; American College of Sports Medicine. American College of Sports Medicine position stand. Quantity and quality of exercise for developing and maintaining cardiorespiratory, musculoskeletal, and neuromotor fitness in apparently healthy adults: guidance for prescribing exercise. Med Sci Sports Exerc. 2011 Jul;43(7):1334-59

Glazer NL, Lyass A, Esliger DW, Blease SJ, Freedson PS, Massaro JM, Murabito JM, Vasan RS. Sustained and shorter bouts of physical activity are related to cardiovascular health. Med Sci Sports Exerc. 2013 Jan;45(1):109-15

Goodwin ML. Blood glucose regulation during prolonged, submaximal, continuous exercise: a guide for clinicians. J Diabetes Sci Technol. 2010 May 1;4(3):694-705

Groppel J. Organizations in motion. Press release from http://corporateathleteedge.com.

Hopkins M, King NA, Blundell JE. Acute and long-term effects of exercise on appetite control: is there any benefit for weight control? Curr Opin Clin Nutr Metab Care. 2010 Nov;13(6):635-40

Katzmarzyk PT, Church TS, Craig CL, Bouchard C. Sitting time and mortality from all causes, cardiovascular disease, and cancer. Med Sci Sports Exerc. 2009 May;41(5):998-1005

Lakerveld J, Dunstan D, Bot S, Salmon J, Dekker J, Nijpels G, Owen N. Abdominal obesity, TV-viewing time and prospective declines in physical activity. Prev Med. 2011 Oct;53(4-5):299-302

Levine JA, Vander Weg MW, Hill JO, Klesges RC. Non-exercise activity thermogenesis: the crouching tiger hidden dragon of societal weight gain. Arterioscler Thromb Vasc Biol. 2006 Apr;26(4):729-36

Levine JA, Miller JM. The energy expenditure of using a "walk-and-work" desk for office workers with obesity. Br J Sports Med. 2007 Sep;41(9):558-61

Marks BL, Katz LM, Smith JK. Exercise and the aging mind: buffing the baby boomer's body and brain. Phys Sportsmed. 2009 Apr;37(1):119-25

Martins C, Morgan L, Truby H. A review of the effects of exercise on appetite regulation: an obesity perspective. Int J Obes (Lond). 2008 Sep;32(9):1337-47

Martin CK, Church TS, Thompson AM, Earnest CP, Blair SN. Exercise dose and quality of life: a randomized controlled trial. Arch Intern Med. 2009 Feb 9;169(3):269-78

Mikus CR, Oberlin DJ, Libla JL, Taylor AM, Booth FW, Thyfault JP. Lowering physical activity impairs glycemic control in healthy volunteers. Med Sci Sports Exerc. 2012 Feb;44(2):225-31

Reaven GM. Insulin resistance: the link between obesity and cardiovascular disease. Med Clin North Am. 2011 Sep;95(5):875-92

Redman LM, Heilbronn LK, Martin CK, de Jonge L, Williamson DA, Delany JP, Ravussin E; Pennington CALERIE Team. Metabolic and behavioral compensations in response to caloric restriction: implications for the maintenance of weight loss. PLoS One. 2009;4(2):e4377

Sim AY, Wallman KE, Fairchild TJ, Guelfi KJ. High-intensity intermittent exercise attenuates ad-libitum energy intake. Int J Obes (Lond). 2013 Jun 4

Thorp AA, Owen N, Neuhaus M, Dunstan DW. Sedentary behaviors and subsequent health outcomes in adults a systematic review of longitudinal studies, 1996-2011. Am J Prev Med. 2011 Aug;41(2):207-15

Tikkanen O, Haakana P, Pesola AJ, Häkkinen K, Rantalainen T, Havu M, Pullinen T, Finni T. Muscle activity and inactivity periods during normal daily life. PLoS One. 2013;8(1):e52228

van der Ploeg HP, Chey T, Korda RJ, Banks E, Bauman A. Sitting time and all-cause mortality risk in 222 497 Australian adults. Arch Intern Med. 2012 Mar 26;172(6):494-500

Voss MW, Prakash RS, Erickson KI, Basak C, Chaddock L, Kim JS, Alves H, Heo S, Szabo AN, White SM, Wójcicki TR, Mailey EL, Gothe N, Olson EA, McAuley E, Kramer AF. Plasticity of brain networks in a randomized intervention trial of exercise training in older adults. Front Aging Neurosci. 2010;2

Wen CP, Wai JP, Tsai MK, Yang YC, Cheng TY, Lee MC, Chan HT, Tsao CK, Tsai SP, Wu X. Minimum amount of physical activity for reduced mortality and extended life expectancy: a prospective cohort study. Lancet. 2011 Oct 1;378(9798):1244-53

Werle CO, Wansink B, Payne CR. Just thinking about exercise makes me serve more food. Physical activity and calorie compensation. Appetite. 2011 Apr;56(2):332-5

Williams PT. Greater weight loss from running than walking during a 6.2-yr prospective follow-up. Med Sci Sports Exerc. 2013 Apr;45(4):706-13

Wilmot EG, Edwardson CL, Achana FA, Davies MJ, Gorely T, Gray LJ, Khunti K, Yates T, Biddle SJ. Sedentary time in adults and the association with diabetes, cardiovascular disease and death: systematic review and meta-analysis. Diabetologia. 2012 Nov;55(11):2895-905

Chapter 13: Refueling Around Movement

Ainsworth BE, Haskell WL, Herrmann SD, Meckes N, Bassett DR Jr, Tudor-Locke C, Greer JL, Vezina J, Whitt-Glover MC, Leon AS. 2011 Compendium of Physical Activities: a second update of codes and MET values. Med Sci Sports Exerc. 2011 Aug;43(8):1575-81

Beelen M, Burke LM, Gibala MJ, van Loon L JC. Nutritional strategies to promote postexercise recovery. Int J Sport Nutr Exerc Metab. 2010 Dec;20(6):515-32

Blom PC, Vøllestad NK, Costill DL. Factors affecting changes in muscle glycogen concentration during and after prolonged exercise. Acta Physiol Scand Suppl. 1986;556:67-74

Bohé J, Low A, Wolfe RR, Rennie MJ. Human muscle protein synthesis is modulated by extracellular, not intramuscular amino acid availability: a dose-response study. J Physiol. 2003 Oct 1;552(Pt 1):315-24

Churchward-Venne TA, Burd NA, Phillips SM. Nutritional regulation of muscle protein synthesis with resistance exercise: strategies to enhance anabolism. Nutr Metab (Lond). 2012 May 17;9(1):40

Colombani PC, Mannhart C, Mettler S. Carbohydrates and exercise performance in non-fasted athletes: a systematic review of studies mimicking real-life. Nutr J. 2013 Jan 28;12:16

Coyle EF, Coggan AR, Hemmert MK, Ivy JL. Muscle glycogen utilization during prolonged strenuous exercise when fed carbohydrate. J Appl Physiol (1985). 1986 Jul;61(1):165-72

Gonzalez JT, Veasey RC, Rumbold PL, Stevenson EJ. Breakfast and exercise contingently affect postprandial metabolism and energy balance in physically active males. Br J Nutr. 2013 Aug;110(4):721-32

Howarth KR, Moreau NA, Phillips SM, Gibala MJ. Coingestion of protein with carbohydrate during recovery from endurance exercise stimulates skeletal muscle protein synthesis in humans. J Appl Physiol (1985). 2009 Apr;106(4):1394-402

Jensen TE, Richter EA. Regulation of glucose and glycogen metabolism during and after exercise. J Physiol. 2012 Mar 1;590(Pt 5):1069-76

Kerksick C, Harvey T, Stout J, Campbell B, Wilborn C, Kreider R, Kalman D, Ziegenfuss T, Lopez H, Landis J, Ivy JL, Antonio J. International Society of Sports Nutrition position stand: nutrient timing. J Int Soc Sports Nutr. 2008 Oct 3;5:17

Moore DR, Areta J, Coffey VG, Stellingwerff T, Phillips SM, Burke LM, Cléroux M, Godin JP, Hawley JA. Daytime pattern of post-exercise protein intake affects whole-body protein turnover in resistance-trained males. Nutr Metab (Lond). 2012 Oct 16;9(1):91

O'Reilly J, Wong SH, Chen Y. Glycaemic index, glycaemic load and exercise performance. Sports Med. 2010 Jan 1;40(1):27-39

Tipton KD, Rasmussen BB, Miller SL, Wolf SE, Owens-Stovall SK, Petrini BE, Wolfe RR. Timing of amino acid-carbohydrate ingestion alters anabolic response of muscle to resistance exercise. Am J Physiol Endocrinol Metab. 2001 Aug;281(2):E197-206

About Dr. Jo

Dr. Jo® is an accomplished author, speaker, freelance writer, and media spokesperson who inspires busy people to stay healthy, sane, and productive. Dr. Jo® has appeared on 300+ TV and radio shows, presented more than 1000 programs at conferences, and has written articles or has been quoted in 300+ newspapers, magazines, and websites. She also serves as a media spokesperson for major companies and is the author of four books.

As a proven, professional speaker, Dr. Jo® is recognized for her energy, humor and audience participation. Dr. Jo® has presented more than 1000 programs to a wide variety of companies and conferences in North America including Compaq/HP, AT&T, Exxon/Mobil, Marriott, Hyatt, US Border Patrol, IBM, Speaking of Women's Health, National Association of Professional Organizers, Restaurants & Institutions Summit, and the National Wellness Conference. She offers plenty of real-life, practical advice that even the busiest of people can incorporate into their lives. Topics include Reboot: how to stay focused, energized, and more productive; How to Stay Healthy & Fit on the Road; What Every Woman Wants: great legs, more energy, & peace of mind; and Swimming in a Sea of Priorities. Dr. Jo® also trains business executives on how to manage their energy through Human Performance Institute (a Johnson & Johnson company).

As president of her own company for more than 20 years, Jo has touched millions of people through her books, articles, and the mass media. Dr. Jo® has served as a media spokesperson for companies including CanolaInfo, Starbucks, Benefiber, Burger King, NutriGrain, NatureMade, Yoplait, SlimFast, Trident, and Wendy's. She has appeared on more than 300 radio and TV shows including CNN, The Daily Buzz, Daytime TV, and the Fox News Channel. Her quotes and articles have appeared in 300+ newspapers, magazines, and websites including the Washington Post, USA Today, Business Traveler, NorthWest Airlines World Traveler, Muscle & Fitness, Fit, Women's World, Prevention, Cooking Light, and USATODAY.com. Her books include Eat Out Healthy, How to Stay Healthy & Fit on the Road, and Dr. Jo's No Big Deal Diet.

Dr. Jo®, a registered dietitian, earned her bachelors (SUNY) and master's degree (Virginia Polytechnic Institute) in nutrition and began her career as a clinical dietitian. At the age of 26 she founded the four-year accredited dietetics program at the University of Texas/Pan American. Dr. Jo® earned her Ph.D. in adult education from Texas A&M University researching the difficult issue of how to help people make healthy changes in all aspects of their lives.

Dr. Jo® practices what she preaches – eating mostly healthy foods on a regular basis, along with a bit of chocolate and diet coke. She and her husband enjoy ballroom dancing, yoga, kayaking, running, skiing, and surfing. And, every Wednesday night you'll catch her on the dance floor tap dancing!

Connect with Dr. Jo:

- www.DrJo.com (videos, articles, and more)

- www.Facebook.com/GoDrJo (what's new with Dr. Jo and RE-BOOT)

- www.Twitter.com/GoDrJo (daily tips related to health and energy)

- www.Pinterest.com/GoDrJo (posting meal and snack ideas, suggestions for dining out, motivational quotes, and more

- Dr. Jo's email newsletter: To sign up, text DRJO to 22828

To book Dr. Jo® to speak to your group or to purchase RE-BOOT in quantity, email your request to AskMe@DrJo.com.

CPSIA information can be obtained
at www.ICGtesting.com
Printed in the USA
LVOW04s0610160916

504888LV00001B/2/P